NAVIGATING
TO VALUE
IN HEALTHCARE

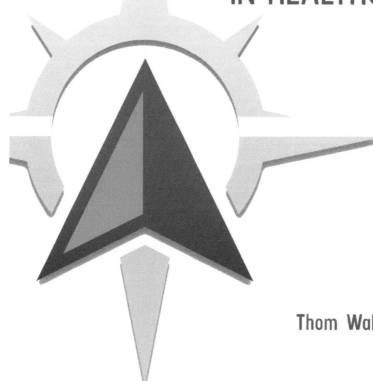

Thom Walsh, PhD

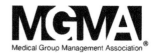
Medical Group Management Association®

NAVIGATING
TO VALUE
IN HEALTHCARE

THOM WALSH

Library of Congress Cataloging-in-Publication Data
Walsh, Thomas
MGMA (Association); publisher.
EGZ Publications; production.
Navigating to Greater Value in Healthcare
 p ; cm
Includes bibliographical references.

Description: 1st. | Englewood, CO : Medical Group Management Association,
 Thomas Walsh.
 c2017. | Includes bibliographical references.

Subjects: 1. Medical care-U.S.-Marketing 2. Medicine-Practice-U.S.-Management [DNLM 1. Management of Health Services-Methods-U.S. 2. Practice Management, Medical-U.S.]

MGMA product id 9051

PRINT ISBN 978-1- 56829-530- 5

Praise for Navigating to Value in Healthcare

"Dr. Thom Walsh has approached this landscape of healthcare reform and its associated stresses as an innovator seizing an opportunity. His very practical perspective has been used by both our individual providers and the administrators of our group practice. In this book, he answers the question, "what can I/we do that will lead to meaningful impact for the patients and the practice?"

His answer lies in designing care that includes the capacity to measure what matters most to patients, learn from the measurements, and to make changes needed to improve the measures while also being mindful of costs. This book helps all of us to define, measure, execute change, and continually improve value for the patients.

From working with Thom, we have come to believe the challenges of payment reform provide us with an opportunity because providers and organizations that consistently deliver value will have a competitive advantage."

~Geoff McCullen MD, MS,
Orthopedic Surgeon

"Walsh's unique perspective arises from his wide-ranging experience innovating across healthcare disciplines… 25 years that extends from front-line service delivery to path breaking scholarship. This book is hard hitting and imminently practical."

~Chris Trimble,
Adjunct Professor, Dartmouth College,
Author of six books on innovation

"In an uncertain landscape, Walsh equips healthcare leaders with a map, a flashlight, and courage. The map points at the power of expertise and data already available for most healthcare organizations. The flashlight uses the latest science of healthcare delivery to illuminate how to learn from variability, improve quality, and enhance value to patients. Leaders will also learn from Dr. Walsh's courageous example of holding fast to his true north of careful and kind care for all."

~Victor M. Montori, MD, MSc,
Professor of Medicine, Mayo Clinic and Chairman, The Patient Revolution

"*The knowledge and experience Dr. Walsh shares in Navigating to Value has proven to be invaluable to our independent physician organization. With his help, our administrators have become convinced that better value is better business and our physicians have become more integrated. We are a stronger and more cohesive group with this knowledge and more confident in our ability to move forward during this era of rapid change.*"

~ Ryan Bohy,
Executive Director of OneHealth Nebraska

"*With everyone talking about healthcare value and transformation it is easy to find so-called experts giving advice, but very few of those experts have actually used outcome measures that matter to patients and made changes to an organization based on results. Dr. Walsh's book connects the realities and challenges of delivering healthcare today with the organizational change theories the experts like to write about. Each chapter gives practical tools that will help you make meaningful change tomorrow. Written by someone who has done it, this is a must read for anyone wanting to do more than just talk about better value.*"

~ Doug Salvador, MD, MPH,
Vice President of Medical Affairs, Baystate Medical Center

TABLE OF CONTENTS

FOREWARD

Oklahoma has never scored particularly well on health or prosperity indicators. Along with our brethren in Arkansas, Kentucky, Louisiana, and Mississippi, we've been banished for decades to the 'bad kids' corner on many measures of prosperity, health, and social well-being. Although our citizens and policymakers annually decry these results, little has seemed to change – the trajectory marched steadily downward. Even across less challenged states and communities, a vicious cycle continues to threaten prosperity: healthcare is becoming so expensive it limits investments in other areas of the economy. Nowhere is this felt more acutely than at the municipal level, where rising healthcare spending limits investments in infrastructure, education, and public safety. Fewer roads, schools, and police and fire personnel mean fewer local jobs, which in turn diminishes tax revenues and further inhibits those citizens' ability to afford healthcare services.

Cutting healthcare costs without regard for the cuts effect on outcomes and coverage is unacceptable. A better approach is required – one that simultaneously improves outcomes and expands coverage, while being mindful of costs.

Dr. Thom Walsh takes us on a journey that closely examines what is required to create greater value in healthcare. Specifically, he bridges the gap between what academics recommend from their research, and what doers are practically accomplishing on the ground. Both are charged with creating better value for patients across the health delivery system. But bridging the gap requires new skills, ethical leadership, and change management. With that perspective in mind, many healthcare executives are going back to school – taking courses that address variation in the delivery of care, cost allocation methods, ethics, leadership, and change management. As a visiting scholar in the University of Tulsa Health Care Delivery Sciences program, Dr. Walsh has taught and mentored our students – those who are charged with reversing Oklahoma's negative trends. In Navigating to Value, Walsh provides colorful and practical examples of ways that health delivery systems can collaborate with their host communities, providing better value to both patients and providers of health care alike. He cites cases in which the system fails, but later succeeds in addressing patients with chronic medical and social conditions. As an example, we meet a man with chronic disabling back pain, who also struggles with diabetes, a learning disability, an addiction, and co-morbid depression. We learned how integration and collaboration between the healthcare delivery system and community are needed to offer him the care he needs.

Tulsa's story is important because history confirms what the pioneering healthcare delivery systems are reporting back as they have launched efforts to improve the value of their care. The pioneering systems have been telling us that greater collaboration is required between the delivery system and the community it serves. In 2006, The University of Oklahoma School of Public Health reported a fourteen-year difference in life expectancy across several neighborhoods of our city, some less than five miles apart. With the release of the study, a "moral outrage" spread across the community. The outrage sparked a litany of public-private partnerships, philanthropic outpouring, and new city-county level efforts. Over the ensuing decade, poverty rates and income inequality have grown worse, yet life expectancy in Tulsa's poorest neighborhoods actually improved. While the progress may be slow, Oklahoma's needle is slowly beginning to move in the right direction. Our progress did not come until we began asking our patients what mattered most (to borrow one of Dr. Walsh's phrases), collaborating with them, and better integrating our efforts with theirs. Our progress started when we began physically locating clinics and physicians in disadvantaged neighborhoods, focusing on the social determinates of health, and building key relationships with community stakeholders. Then fourteen-year difference in life expectancy began to shrink. The difference is now eleven years. While this is still too high, the improvement is a feat no other American city has replicated.

The Tulsa experience taught us that relationships matter. Collaboration and integration between patients and providers as well as the medical and social-services sectors have been keys to unlocking success. To strengthen relationships and truly build partnerships, we carefully listened to the people we serve. In other words, we adopted what Dr. Walsh outlines in this book: identifying what matters most to patients, measuring what matters in order to create care plans, and using the data to inform our strategic thinking as we craft partnerships. We now include patients and stakeholders from the community to help design new facilities and systems of care. We hire staff and providers that live in the neighborhood. And we are honest when regarding our past mistakes, especially when trying to improve quality, expand access, and contain costs – thus breaking the vicious cycle described above.

Our solutions may not effectively translate to every community – no single overarching model will revolutionize healthcare. But in his narrative, Dr. Walsh describes ways to create a capacity for measuring what matters most to patients. He shows us how to increase the value of care, and ways of reengineering the health system of the future. By adapting these lessons, it is likely you will identify your own local and community-based solutions.

by

Gerald P. Clancy MD,
President, Tulsa University

&

Jeffrey S. Alderman MD, MS,
Director, TU Institute for Health Care Delivery Sciences, Associate Professor, Community Medicine, Tulsa University

CHAPTER 1

BUILDING VALUE INTO HEALTHCARE DELIVERY

INTRODUCTION: CREATING GREATER VALUE IN HEALTHCARE

This book is about creating greater value in healthcare. It is one thing to understand the concept of value; it is another to know what needs to change in an organization and how to get it done. This includes moving an organization to a place where all of its leaders are not only aware of financial performance, but also aware of outcomes that matter to patients as well as how the quantity and quality of their services compare to similar organizations. Beyond awareness, leaders need new types of information, knowledge, and skills in order to act quickly and to successfully improve underperforming areas.

This type of organizational agility is necessary because there are many changes happening currently in healthcare payment reform. Since the 1960s there have been major revisions to Medicare and Medicaid every decade or so, and we should expect changes to continue. Recent examples include Value-Based Payments to hospital systems and the Medicare Access and CHIP Reauthorization Act and its Merit-based Incentive Payment System (MIPS). In this book, I will not attempt to go into detail about the nuances of these emerging and evolving trends because I believe a book of that type will have a very short shelf life. Rather I will describe an approach to delivering healthcare that has been successfully used for over 20 years in an academic medical center, independent physician offices, and is now being implemented in a military medical facility. Knowing what matters most to patients, and systematically trying to improve those outcomes, while maintaining or lowering the costs it takes to achieve those outcomes, is not only better value, it is better business. This is true no matter the political, regulatory, or payment environment.

For example, one day 25 years ago, as I sat at talking at lunch with my colleagues, I was wondering what I had gotten myself into. I had little more than a year of experience in a small group private practice as an orthopedic physical therapist, and the two senior therapists were nervous. I was struggling to take in some unfamiliar terms, such as *payment reform, capitation, preferred provider status*, and the strangest one of all—the proposed Health Security Act of 1993, colloquially known as the Clinton Health Plan. It was the earlier 1990s and my colleagues had me convinced we would all lose our shirts as the practice buckled under new regulations.

My lack of familiarity with the issues being discussed added to my unease, and I left the lunch feeling as though my livelihood was forever threatened. Having grown up in a single-parent home in a small village nestled between Lake Ontario and the Adirondack Mountains in Northern New York State, I was the first in my family to go to college. I had left my mother and sister with a mixture of uncertainty and guilt. I didn't know anyone who had gone to college. I felt guilty about leaving my family, but I convinced myself that a college education would enable me to be a better son, brother, husband and one day, a father. Now the Clinton Health Plan, as I understood it at the time, meant severe limitations on my earnings and possibly even the viability of our practice.

Over several weeks we launched a plan. We believed our practice was the best in the region. We even said so in our yellow pages ad. Truth be told, we had no idea how good we were or how we compared to any other physical therapy service provider. Our plan was risky, because we were going to take steps to learn how much—or how little—we were helping our patients.

We agreed to start asking our patients about their pain and function at each of their visits on one sheet of paper using three questions about pain and 10 questions about function. We made space on the back of the page to write our notes for the treatment session. We asked the receptionist to hand the sheet of paper to patients when they arrived and we placed it in their charts at the end of the session.

I was nervous because my colleagues had much more experience than me and I was certain my patients' improvement, as measured by the pain and function scores, was not going to as much as theirs I was confident of one thing: No matter how low I scored, I could learn and get better.

My anxiety over my status proved baseless. Our small group found the new information fascinating. Admittedly, we were the only ones looking at the data. We simply observed our patients scores and talked about what we saw on an almost daily basis. We did not let months go by to then aggregate the data and discuss averages. In addition to our internal discussions, we also discussed the data with our patients *as we treated them*. I always made a point to thank each patient for answering the questions. I showed each patient his or her scores and asked clarifying questions. After a few weeks, I started carving out time on nights and weekends to enter de-identified data into a spreadsheet, where we captured each patient's diagnosis, initial pain and function scores, the number of treatments approved by the payer, the number of treatments to date, the most recent pain and function scores, and the difference between the initial scores and the most current.

We learned a lot over the weeks and months that followed. For example, patients loved it when we talked with them about their scores as we took their history and during follow-up visits. Patterns emerged from the functional data: For example, a patient under 60 years old with back and leg pain to his foot who felt worse in the morning and better as the day progressed, worse sitting, lifting, or bending repeatedly and better on the move, walking, or lying down, most likely had one diagnosis, and would respond well to a specific regimen of exercise. On the other hand, an older patient with leg pain made worse by walking and relieved by sitting had, most likely, one of two diagnoses. One diagnosis was mechanical, related to her back, and something I could help, while the other was vascular and something I could not easily affect. The key to distinguishing the difference between the two was to ask, "Help me understand the trouble you're having walking; are your symptoms better or worse if you are going uphill, or does the incline make no difference? Symptoms made worse with uphill walking are more likely to be vascular. In this way, the patient-reported information helped me to diagnosis and care for the individual in front of me at that specific visit.

By using this type of information, we began to develop an ability to discern who was likely to respond to our care, who would not, and to estimate how many sessions a responder would require. Most providers develop this intuition over time, but we could now quantify it.

After several more months, our patient charts were getting thick, my colleagues and I were feeling confident and wanted to show off our efforts. We hosted an evening seminar for local representatives from the region's commercial payers. There was some cheese, a little wine, and I used an overhead projector to show our data collection form. I also displayed several completed forms that I had de-identified. I was able to share that my average patient was 48 years old, entered treatment with pain scores slightly over 8 out of 10, where 10 is the worst imaginable, and function scores in the low 20s out of 100, where 100 is normal function. At discharge, average pain scores were below two and function scores were over 85. In addition, these changes were happening over a series of five to six visits while most prescriptions for therapy were written by physicians and then approved by payers for 12 visits. I was, on average, saving the payer the expense of six to seven visits. We explained our plan to use the forms with all of our patients and our plans to provide any requesting payer with the average number of visits and average change score for our most common diagnoses.

Then, we unveiled our reason for the plan—we proposed the payers use data to determine their preferred providers. That is, we wanted them to compare our outcomes to the outcomes produced by other practices in the area. The payer representatives were thrilled by the idea! They also quickly learned that no one else was collecting data. We were granted preferred status, essentially by default. No one ever asked to review any of the data we collected.

We believed the decision to start asking patients about their pain and function was central to our ability to quickly gain preferred provider status among the region's commercial payers. The patient information also distinguished us to the physicians referring patients to us. The practice grew quickly over the next six years from a single entity in the basement of a medical office building to four practices over a 50-mile radius. Along the way, we learned lessons about the ripple effects created by changing a practice, where even the simple act of handing a piece of paper to a patient and requesting their participation could create complex downstream effects.

Those days seem like a distant memory, but now, once again, it is a chaotic and uncertain time in the healthcare industry. Payment for healthcare based on the volume of services is phasing out because it has proven to be unsustainable. Meanwhile, new payment methods based on outcomes achieved and quality of service are not fully tested. The challenge of finding a sustainable way to deliver healthcare to all is a difficult one, which makes it tempting to watch, wait and hope that the latest reform effort will pass and "things will get back to normal." They will not. Paying for healthcare has simply gotten too expensive for individuals, businesses and communities. While the rate of growth in healthcare spending has slowed in recent years, paying for healthcare is still among the most common reasons for an individual to declare bankruptcy. It is also still among the largest expenses for employers, and local governments are still struggling with healthcare expenses that cost communities millions of dollars that could be spent on infrastructure, education and safety. Infrastructure and education promote commerce and innovation that are proven pathways toward better standards of living and better health. Lower levels of education and living standards, in turn, are associated with a greater need for healthcare. The realization that delivering healthcare can cure disease, ease suffering, and also financially devastate individuals, businesses and communities, has had a galvanizing effect on our nation. We want to "fix healthcare" even if there is no consensus on how to do it.

While consensus on how to fix healthcare delivery remains elusive, a majority agrees that the way we pay for healthcare had to be changed. Paying healthcare providers based on the volume of services performed contributes to the overuse of diagnostic procedures and treatments. These excesses are costly and can be harmful. An evolving approach is to base payment not on volume, but on the outcomes achieved and the quality of services delivered for each dollar spent. This means that rather than paying a healthcare provider for every clinical encounter with a patient with diabetes—a method that rewards more encounters regardless of benefit or harm to the patient—healthcare providers would be paid based on the rate of avoidable amputations in this patient population and the quality of the care experience as reported by the patients. This method rewards outcomes and service. It does not limit the volume of clinical encounters to those who need each one, but it does incentivize fewer encounters whenever possible. More simply, payment systems are transitioning from volume- to value-based. For healthcare leaders, this means the future will require an ability to know the outcomes your healthcare system is producing, the quality of care experienced by patients, and the costs to produce them. The future will also require agility, as indicated by an ability to rapidly recognize areas that are in need of improvement, to briskly build a sense of common purpose regarding what change must be made, and then to deftly deploy personnel who are experienced in executing the needed changes. In essence, the transformation from volume- to value-based payments for healthcare requires an agile learning organization.

THE NEED FOR DATA

Truly successful improvement and creating greater value require data in order to assess the current situation and monitor the effects of our interventions. Data that provide insight into both what matters most to patients and the costs of providing care can be difficult to find. Medical outcomes like "survival" are meaningful, but very blunt, and not nearly nuanced enough for the task of improving how healthcare is delivered. Other medically important data like A1C levels among patients with diabetes, provide insight for clinicians, but are cryptic and lack meaning for the individuals with the condition. Creating greater value also requires leaders to be informed and knowledgeable of the costs associated with delivering care. Even here, old methods are changing and new skills are needed. Cost accounting is relatively simple if calculations include only doctors' salaries and supplies, but complex if you intend to allocate administrators, support staff and infrastructure as well. Simply put, healthcare, like other industries, is transforming in a way that is increasingly reliant on data. The right data, along with the skills needed to turn the data into useful information and to build knowledge, can be difficult, and for many, impossible to find.

Finding the data necessary for leading a high-value and agile healthcare delivery system is only part of the battle. The needed data, when they do exist, are kept in multiple databases that were built for privacy, not for sharing. The data need to be retrieved, organized and displayed in ways that inform and enable decisive action.

Leadership is crucial for decisive action to succeed. However, even a well-informed leader is not enough. Healthcare delivery occurs in teams. Leaders must build a vision that outlines an inspiring future for their organizations, and identify an achievable first step to build momentum and overcome the resistance to change that lurks in all humans and organizations.

The ability to learn from prior efforts and to execute changes with agility has not been a hallmark of the existing healthcare industry. Today's chaotic environment requires all of this to happen much more quickly than before. A few organizations have been building their ability to create value, learn quickly and execute successfully for some time. They have created a checklist of essential ingredients for anyone starting now (Table 1).

TABLE 1.1: A CEO's CHECKLIST FOR HIGH-VALUE CARE		
Foundational Elements	1.	Governance priority (visible and determined leadership by CEO and board)
	2.	Culture of continuous improvement (commitment to ongoing, real-time learning)
Infrastructure Fundamentals	3.	IT best practices (automated, reliable information to and from the point of care)
	4.	Evidence protocols (effective, efficient and consistent care)
	5.	Resource utilization (optimized use of personnel, physical space and other resources)
Care Delivery Priorities	6.	Integrated care (right care, setting, providers and teamwork)
	7.	Shared decision making (patient – provider collaboration)
	8.	Targeted services (tailored to resource intensive patients)
Reliability and Feedback	9.	Embedded safeguards (supports and prompts to reduce injury and infection)
	10.	Internal transparency (visible progression on performance, outcomes and costs)

Cosgrove D, et.al. A CEO checklist for high-value health care. Institute of Medicine. Washington DC 2012.

The checklist outlines the features of an organization built to thrive in any payment system. It is helpful because there is wide variation in how organizations are structured and governed. Some focus solely on care delivery priorities (items 6 through 8 on the CEO checklist). Their thought leaders do an excellent job of describing how a high-value healthcare system would function, in theory. Nevertheless, these leaders often lack the foundational elements and infrastructure fundamentals needed to successfully act on the theories or measure the impact of changes to care-delivery processes. Other organizations are lured by the infrastructure, technology, and data, as if the act of simply providing data to busy healthcare professionals will inspire successful corrective action. These organizations lack the delivery priorities and foundational elements needed to move from data, to insight, and on to action. Strangely, many leaders in these organizations find themselves in a rut as they seek more and more data to inform the next action. Still other organizations have outstanding foundational elements, including excellent leaders with bright minds and hearts in the right places, but they cannot execute needed changes in delivery processes or measure the impact of efforts. They end up fleeting from one improvement method to another, always underachieving. Their leaders' optimism regarding the latest improvement science has to offer, in the face of recalcitrant struggles, breeds cynicism throughout the organization. This is not meant to be an exhaustive typology of healthcare organizational behavior, rather it is meant to show that transforming an organization to create value requires a full complement of leadership, data, knowledge of how to use the data, and an ability to learn as they go.

Many leaders say their organizations prioritize the delivery of high-value care, but few measure how well they are doing. Indeed, a broad survey of U.S. hospitals found just 32% of hospital boards received any formal training in care delivery and quality improvement, and only 20% of respondents reported that its chairperson, the board itself, or one of its committees was an influential force for improving quality throughout their hospitals. Regardless of how highly an organization prioritized quality, awareness of how well their organization's quality fared compared to others was poor. Nationally, 66% of hospital board chairs rated the quality of care at their organizations as better, or much better, than average. Among low-performing hospitals, none rated their organizations as worse, or much worse, than average. Irrespective of categories, approximately 1 of 5 leaders said they did not know how their hospital's quality compared to national means.

FIGURE 1.1: HOSPITAL BOARD CHAIR PERCEPTION OF HOSPITAL PERFORMANCE

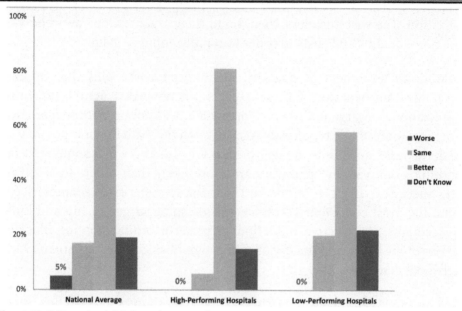

Jha, A.K. & Epstein, A.M. (2009) Hospital governance and the quality of care. *Health Affairs.*
doi: 10.1377/hlthaff.2009.0297

These findings point to opportunities for raising awareness about quality. The opportunities are challenging because, as the same research article makes clear, many leaders do not see optimizing quality or value as a top priority. Indeed, half of all hospital boards did not rate care quality as a top priority for the board or a top metric for assessing CEO performance. Low-performing hospitals, in particular, were more likely to spend their meetings focused on financial performance and were less likely to have a committee review quality metrics and prioritize improvement efforts. Even among hospitals recognizing the need to focus on the value of care, only 20% felt that their governance board was one of the most influential factors determining performance quality.

Awareness of quality is necessary, but not sufficient. Ultimately, leaders must build an organization's capacity to execute the changes necessary to produce high-quality outcomes while also managing the costs associated with the efforts. The ability to successfully execute improvement efforts while also reducing costs is the definition of an agile, learning, and thriving healthcare organization. A high-value, agile learning organization has the awareness and the ability to execute regardless of the latest efforts by politicians to reform the industry or a payment organization's efforts to throttle back utilization. The wisest leaders, then, build their organization's awareness of outcomes, quality, and costs in order to rapidly enhance value.

Building an awareness of quantity, quality and costs, plus the capacity to rapidly improve any of these aspects when needed across an entire organization, are gargantuan tasks. Fortunately, we know from the experience of organizations that have already started down this path that it is possible to break the tasks down into smaller pieces. We also know that some medical conditions or treatment pathways are more likely than others to result in early successes. The conditions and pathways where early adaptors have found the most consistent successes include spine surgeries, hip and knee replacements, the elective induction of preterm births, stenting blocked arteries of the heart, and the use of concurrent hospice care for patients with a terminal diagnosis.

Most hospitals can review publicly available data sources to learn how their quantity and quality compare to best in class or regional competitors for the procedures noted above. Gathering this information provides a vision for what future care can look like. It is also possible to consult the evidence base to learn best practices for these conditions and procedures, but blindly attempting to follow the evidence without consideration for local context and culture is a formula for frustration and disappointment. Discussion and consensus building are required among an organization's leaders and managers to marry local context to the evidence. Trial and error are required as an organization implements new processes. Some will work and some will not. Each subsequent effort builds on lessons learned from the earlier struggles and successes. Using a scientific approach to minimize the influence of chance, bias, and confounding factors in order to assess the impact of improvement efforts leads to organizational wisdom, as well as generating momentum when the ingredients for success are incorporated into the policies and procedures throughout the organization.

Whether you are starting with spine surgeries, hip and knee replacements, the elective induction of preterm births, stenting blocked arteries of the heart, the use of concurrent hospice care for patients with a terminal diagnosis, or another medical condition or procedure, this book is meant to guide an organization through the process of building its capacity to thrive by creating value.

Chapter 2 starts us off with addressing the variation in healthcare delivery. The concept of unwarranted variation in healthcare delivery originated in Scotland with J. Alison Glover, in the 1930s. He found wide variation in the rates of tonsillectomies among Scottish children, with some regions having rates over five times higher than others with no discernable benefit to the children. Indeed, the possibility of harm loomed large as more children died in 1935 from surgical complications than from untended inflammation. Following the Second World War, Jack Wennberg from Dartmouth College picked up the investigation of variation in the delivery of healthcare. This chapter highlights the history of variation research and details how implications from the research can be harnessed in order to drive the organizational changes needed today.

Chapter 3 continues the journey toward measuring real value by showing where to look for value opportunities in the organization. We measure many things in healthcare, but we do not measure value particularly well. That process begins by understanding your data. The chapter begins by presenting the insights available from public data sources. These data form the basis of comparative analyses that can help an organization prioritize its improvement efforts and speed up the overall transformation process. Additional aspects of measurement, including data management, warehouses, registries, and practical considerations regarding collecting, retrieving, organizing and displaying are also presented.

In Chapter 4, we get into the meat of measuring value. Harnessing variation requires much more than just raw data. Measurement must be timely and relevant if you want to increase value. Organizations are in for a painful shock if they believe transformation will happen only due to increased data availability. In fact, experience shows that merely dropping data into a clinical setting will incite a near riotous revolt, breed cynicism, and increase resistance to change. We measure value by assessing outcomes that matter to patients, the quality of their care experience, and the costs required to achieve them. The chapter concludes with a description of how to use "outcome data" at the initial point of care to assist with the intake, triage and navigation of a patient through the care process. In this manner, the traditional thinking about data providing quarterly or yearly feedback is turned on its head. Instead, the data are fed forward to assist the patient and his or her care team in creating greater value now.

We then move on to creating greater value through implementation efforts in Chapter 5. Regardless of whether an improvement idea comes from the ground up or board down, microsystems will implement the idea. Microsystems are present in every healthcare organization right now, even though many within the organization may not realize it. A microsystem consists of a patient, data about the patient and the care team, plus two to eight healthcare workers ranging from receptionists to surgeons. Microsystems form and dissolve organically depending on the patient's needs. This chapter addresses how to recognize a microsystem, how to map a process of care, and the questions to ask that will help inform improvement efforts.

Assessing the impact of transformation efforts, and thereby demonstrating value, is the topic of Chapter 6. Many impact-assessment methods produce erroneous conclusions due to unmeasured variables. The best way to eliminate unmeasured variable bias is through randomization, but that is rarely practical outside of academic settings. For this reason, we cover a more practical approach for dealing with the influence of unmeasured variables— the difference-in-differences method. From there, attention turns to an overview of techniques for monitoring change while it is occurring. These include process control charts for means, proportions, and rare events.

Chapter 7 describes a communication plan and the typical phases of a transformation effort in healthcare. It is possible to think of transformation as a series of improvement efforts, not necessarily in parallel or sequentially, but synergistically with lessons learned being transferred across departmental and project-specific silos. A communication plan is required because a failure to consider who needs to know—and who needs to be involved—in a transformation effort will derail progress. With forethought, it is possible to avoid these obstacles. It is helpful to operationalize the phases of a project because, when done well, it helps guide your organization in the right direction. A good communication plan helps everyone see where things are going and what is required today.

When people define innovation today they most often think of technology infrastructure, big data and new devices, drugs and surgical techniques. They often discount the potential effectiveness of people and teams, and their ability to induce significant improvement and positive change in systems. Chapter 8 begins by describing the attributes of individuals, teams, and organizations that have conducted successful transformation efforts. This is broken down into effective attributes of project teams, project leadership, organizational leadership, organizational support, and mindset and expectations.

Chapter 9 is devoted to explaining transformation efforts known to improve the value of care delivery. A cookbook approach would say, "Apply these liberally to processes involving patients facing spine surgeries, hip or knee replacements, stents for coronary artery disease, early elective induction, and concurrent hospice." The first topic is "hotspotting," which involves identifying the least healthy patients for a clinical condition in order to focus efforts on preventing those very sick patients from getting worse. Some organizations are spending a lot of money to purchase tools to help clinicians identify patients at the highest risk of becoming hospitalized or incurring great costs. Leaders of those organizations should not forget their most valuable hotspotting resource—their own nurses. Ask any nurse to identify the sickest patients most at risk and the patients that require the most intensive management and you'll quickly get a written list.

Then next issue in Chapter 9 is integrating behavioral medicine specialists into care pathways. Patients with the greatest disease burden have multiple comorbidities. Co-morbid adjustment disorders such as anxiety and depression, as well as mental illnesses like schizophrenia, can make it difficult for an individual to behave in ways that promote and enable good health. Evidence also tells us that co-morbid adjustment disorders remain under-diagnosed and under-treated. A co-located behavioral health specialist in primary care setting promotes increased recognition of the problem, raises treatment rates, and decreases hospitalizations and readmissions.

The subject of integrating shared decision making into care pathways continues in Chapter 9. Evidence tells us healthcare providers are not skilled at discerning a patient's preferences and frequently make the wrong preference diagnosis, resulting in patients receiving care they would not have chosen had they been fully informed. A patient receiving care that is not aligned with his or her informed preferences is antithetical to creating value. I introduce a three-question patient-reported survey called CollaboRATE, which has been successful in helping to facilitate shared decision-making.

Chapter 9 also addresses specific actions to improve the patient's experience in the healthcare system. These include communication training and improving the coordination between care teams to create excellent handoffs.

The final topic in Chapter 9 is learning collaboratives. The formation of a learning collaborative has repeatedly been shown to produce substantial improvements in the value of care delivered through:

» Improved outcomes that matter to patients

» Aligning patient preferences and care received

» Fewer treatment complications

» Longer life expectancy

» Avoidance of unwanted intensive care

» Decreased costs

Members of a collaborative learn from one another so the speed of transformation increases for all participants. Meanwhile, forming and maintaining a collaborative has never been easier. Internet use is routine, many people are familiar with online collaboration with remote workers, and video conferencing with screen sharing is free. This chapter includes several examples of successful learning collaboratives.

Chapter 10 outlines the challenges ahead in creating value. A single person can make a profound difference in the world, but it is hard to transform healthcare delivery alone. It takes a team and organizational commitment, but a team of senior leaders cannot mandate successful transformation. It requires engaged people at all levels of the organization. Moreover, it requires an organizational appreciation of the road ahead. The road leads to better value for patients, providers, payers, businesses and communities.

Each chapter contains a list of resources for anyone wishing to take a deeper dive in to a topic. This book is not intended to be a textbook, nor is it my intent to be comprehensive. This book is meant to be an overview of the knowledge and skills needed to build an agile learning healthcare organization with the capacity to create greater value so that it can thrive in today's chaos and tomorrow's uncertainty. I hope you refer to it often.

RESOURCES

» The Massachusetts Heath Policy Commission. (2013). *2013 Cost trend report*. http://www.mass.gov/anf/docs/hpc/2013-cost-trends-report-final.pdf

» Government Accountability Office. (April 2013). *State and local governments' fiscal outlook: April 2013 update*. http://www.gao.gov/special.pubs/longterm/state/index.html

» Bradley, E.H., & Taylor L.A., (2013). The American health care paradox: Why spending more is getting us less. *Public Affairs*.

» Welch, H.G., Schwartz, L.M., & Woloshin, S. (2011) *Overdiagnosed: Making people sick in pursuit of health*. Boston: Beacon Press.

» Brownlee, S. (2007). *Overtreated: Why too much medicine is making us sicker and poorer*. New York: Bloomsbury USA.

» Cosgrove, D., et.al. (2012). *A CEO checklist for high value health care*. Washington, DC: Institute of Medicine.

» Jha, A.K., & Epstein, A.M. (2009). Hospital governance and the quality of care. *Health Affairs*. doi: 10.1377/hlthaff.2009.0297

» Green,S.M., Reid, R.J., & Larson, E.B. Implementing the learning health system: From concept to action. *Ann Intern Med*, 157, 207-210

» Goldsmith J., Burns, L.R., Sen, A., & Goldsmith, T. (2015) *Integrated delivery networks: In search of benefits and market effects*. Washington, DC: The National Academy of Social Insurance.

» Smith, M., Saunders, R., Stuckhardt., L., McGinnis, J.M. (2012). *Best care at lower cost: the path to continuously learning health care in America*. Committee on the Learning Health Care System in America. Washington DC: Institute of Medicine.

» Bohmer, R.M.J. (2010). Fixing health care on the front lines. *Harvard Business Review*. 88, 4, 62-69.

» James, B.C., Savitz, L.A. (2011). How Intermountain trimmed health care costs through robust quality improvement efforts. *Health Affairs*, 30(6), 1185-1191.

» Lee, T.H. (2010). Putting the value framework to work. *N Engl J Med.* 363, 2481-3.

» Kaplan, G., G. Bo-Linn, P. Carayon, P. Pronovost, W. Rouse, P. Reid, &. Saunders, R. (2013). *Bringing a systems approach to health.* Discussion Paper, Institute of Medicine and National Academy of Engineering, Washington, DC. http://www.iom.edu/ systemsapproaches

» Porter M.E. (2010). What is value in health care? *N Engl J Med* 363, 2477-81.

» Porter M.E. & Teisberg E.O. (2006). *Redefining health care: creating value-based competition on results.* Boston: Harvard Business Review Press.

CHAPTER 2

HARNESSING VARIATION TO DRIVE VALUE HIGHER

The History and Modern Implications of Variation in the Healthcare Industry

When an organization starts measuring costs, quality, and outcomes that matter to patients, it will soon be confronted by the Glover phenomenon. J. Alison Glover, from Scotland, first described the curious situation of variation in the delivery of healthcare services in 1938. The number of children dying from complications during or immediately after the surgery to remove their tonsils concerned Dr. Glover. No less than 513 deaths occurred during the four-year period of 1931 to 1935, far greater than the 60 children dying from swollen tonsils during the same period. This was difficult to fathom. These numbers tell of a treatment much more deadly than the disease it was supposed to cure.

This finding led Glover to dig deeper. He collected data that included the number of children with tonsillitis, the number who died from the disease, the number of tonsillectomies, and the number of deaths resulting from the procedure. He decided to organize his investigation by school districts because healthcare providers associated with a school made most diagnoses. He also thought more industrialized regions, with their pollution, could have a higher proclivity for childhood illness, so he recorded whether the child lived near a factory. Because some of the school districts were much larger than others, he converted the raw number of children with disease to a rate and did the same for the surgical procedure. He asked how many cases of tonsillitis and how many tonsillectomies were reported for every 100 students in each district. This equalized comparisons between large and small districts.

What he found made no sense to him.

The variation in tonsillectomy rates was extreme, but the rates for tonsillitis were similar. A child with tonsillitis in the school district with the highest rate of procedures was 27 times more likely to have the procedure than a similar child in the lowest rate district. What could explain this? He considered all the usual suspects and found no ready explanation. A family's economic status did not affect a child's access to care because healthcare was funded through the tax system and free of charge at the point of service. Proximity to industry, overcrowding, poverty, climate, and even the efficiency of the school dental service, made no difference in the procedure rates. For every one of these concerns there was a district with a rate at least twice the national average and a matched district with a rate at least one-half the average. More worrisome still, the procedure rate varied from year to year in some districts, yet the frequency of tonsillitis and diagnoses association with inadequate care, ear infections, deafness, and school absenteeism remained steady over time.

Not only were children dying from the procedure, he could find no evidence of benefit from it in high-rate regions, nor evidence of harm resulting from too few procedures in low-rate regions.

He could also foresee the hornet's nest of difficulty that would ensue if he tried to determine which rate was right. He had faith, however, that medical officers, when shown the data, would take it upon themselves to investigate further. Each officer would examine his own rates and adjust his utilization if it was shown to be an outlier. Glover's work was discussed enough in the U.K. during the late 30s that any observed variation in the utilization of care was dubbed the "Glover Phenomenon."

There was little opportunity for the healthcare industry to act upon Glover's findings. The Second World War and its aftermath diverted everyone's attention during the 1940s and 1950s. The Glover phenomenon was noted again in the '60s as countries worked to rebuild their healthcare systems because the variation in utilization of services made it impossible to accurately predict how much infrastructure would be needed in any particular location. The predominant concern was making sure there was adequate care for all.

Immediately following World War II, the United States passed the Hill-Burton Act, which spurred construction of hospitals and the expansion of healthcare services across the country. By the 1960s, policy makers became concerned about illness among the old and those born with or acquiring medical conditions needing medical attention, but having no hopes of employment that would enable them to pay for healthcare. Laws creating Medicare and Medicaid were passed to remedy those concerns. Ensuring adequate access to medical care remained a high priority throughout the decade.

In the 1970s, a physician-researcher came to Northern New England in the United States to determine whether the healthcare needs of the region remained underserved despite Hill-Burton, Medicare and Medicaid. To investigate, Dr. Jack Wennberg gathered data on the prevalence of childhood illnesses and the utilization of hospital services in Vermont. He calculated rates just as Glover had, but instead of organizing his data by school systems, he organized it into regions around hospitals.

Tonsillitis was a frequent diagnosis among children across the state. The illness rate was similar and relatively stable. This was not surprising because air quality and climate were similar for all children in the region. However, the variation in the rate of tonsillectomies was extreme. Indeed, a child in one township could be five to six times more likely to have his tonsils removed than a child in just one town over. Northern New England at the time was very homogenous, almost entirely white, and low to middle income. Neither race nor family income could explain the variation in treatment.

Unknowingly, Wennberg had repeated Glover's analysis, and Wennberg's findings were similar to Glover's. They both found large variation in tonsillectomy rates across relatively small homogenous regions and neither could identify a suitable explanation for so much variation. In this pre-Internet era, Wennberg traveled to each township in order to collect his data. He knew many of the physicians and surgeons by name. He willingly shared his findings with his colleagues and discussed possible explanations.

Mischievously, Wennberg tabled the rate of tonsillitis, tonsillectomies and the change in rates over time for each township, but with the town name removed. He asked his colleagues to pick out their own towns. Not one of them could. The care providers in a region were blind to regional treatment rates. The anonymity in this method invited conversations about causes and remedies instead of rancor and excuses. While no direct and easy answer was found, something did happen during the early days of these discussions: the treatment rates converged. The higher-rate township's rate decreased and the lower-rate township's rate increased, but no surgeon admitted to consciously altering his indications for surgery.

Intrigued, Wennberg continued to extend his analysis to additional diagnoses and treatments. The rate of hip fractures was similar region to region, as was the rate of hospitalization due to the fracture. The rates for illnesses and injuries for almost every other diagnosis were similarly stable, but unlike hip fractures, treatment rates always varied. More interestingly still, one township might have a high rate for one treatment compared to its neighbors, but a low rate for others. No region held the highest rates for all procedures and none held the lowest across the board. Instead, each township seemed to have its own unique profile of rates for common procedures.

Under-treatment remained the primary concern of the time. Wennberg set out to determine the degree to which patients in low-rate regions suffered from the lack of medical care. He found no evidence of suffering. For example, children in the regions where fewer tonsillectomies were performed were no more likely to suffer from deafness, respiratory disease, or even missed school days. Wennberg could find no apparent advantage for the children in the high-rate treatment regions, nor disadvantage for children in the lower-rate regions. The only consistent finding was the higher number of surgical complications in the higher-rate regions. While it was easy to assume that more healthcare was better, Wennberg came to see there was a flip side. Like Glover, who observed more deaths from the operation to treat swollen tonsils than from the condition left untreated, Wennberg saw there was potential benefit from healthcare services, and there was potential harm.

Wennberg next extended his techniques to larger cities. He began by comparing Boston, Massachusetts, and New Haven, Connecticut. Both contained Ivy League universities and had similar demographics. In addition, both liked to market themselves as "the best." Wennberg found each city to have a unique signature of procedures. He found no apparent loss among patients with diagnoses receiving less care and no added gain for patients receiving more care. In addition, he found the providers in Boston and New Haven were similar to those in Vermont in their lack of knowledge about their treatment rates. In fact, when shown unlabeled treatment rates, the providers were unable to identify their own regions.

The Boston/New Haven research occurred in the 1980s. Dr. Wennberg went on to compare top-ranked academic medical centers to one another and the Glover phenomenon held. There is variation in the outcomes, quality and costs associated with the delivery of healthcare services everywhere, even among the institutions that pride themselves in being "the best in the world." In 2013, the Institute of Medicine (now the National Academy of Medicine) issued a report summarizing all the work on variation in the delivery of healthcare, including all of Dr. Wennberg's. The IOM authors concluded that variation in delivery exists at every level of service provision, from large regions to small areas, and even within individual treatment facilities. The variation they found could not be fully explained by differences in the needs or desires of patients, meaning some patients were receiving care they would not have received elsewhere or would not have chosen had they been aware of their options. Moreover, the additional care in some patients were receiving did not confer any additional benefit.

VARIATION AS AN AGENT OF ORGANIZATIONAL CHANGE

The idea that more care is not always better or even necessary is so counterintuitive that most people react to it defensively, with multiple excuses, but another view is possible. The alternative view, based on data showing variation, is that high-value care exists now. Someone somewhere is taking care of patients every bit as sick as the sickest and they are achieving better outcomes, providing better quality service, and they are doing it at lower costs. Instead of being inspired to make excuses, wise leaders are inspired to collaborate, innovate, and adapt.

Whatever you measure in healthcare, whether it is from an external data source like the Dartmouth Atlas or from data sources within your organization, you will find variation. If you plot out the data, you will end up with a distribution. In healthcare, you will not find a normal distribution where the majority of observations are somewhere in the middle. Instead, it is more likely you will find a long tail in one direction. That is, it will be skewed. If you are observing illness severity, most patients will be relatively healthy, but a few will be very, very sick. Similarly, if you are observing readmission rates, most will be low, but those of a few hospitals, clinics, or clinicians will be very high. On the other hand, maybe you are observing patient-reported outcomes for a hospital, a clinic, or a clinician. Most will be somewhere from good to great; a few will be very low.

There is a fear about revealing variation. The fear is that the organizations or individuals will be ranked, and then those in the bad tail of the skewed distribution will be spanked. That is, underperformers will be called out, and somehow punished. Worse still, many leaders do not prepare their organizations for the data release, which inevitably leads to worries about the methods for collecting, retrieving, organizing, and displaying the data. This breeds hostility because to each person being assessed, it feels like he or she is being unknowingly evaluated, and no one takes kindly to pop-up exams.

If you want to build an organization that is fearful, angry, cynical, and full of resistance to change, dump in data without explanation and start ranking and spanking.

If you want an agile learning organization that transforms to meet the needs of the people it serves, you will want to harness variation and use it to create greater value.

What are the keys to harnessing variation? First, before any data are released, build shared knowledge, shared language, and mutual respect among the people who could be impacted by it. Explain that you are building a learning organization, not a blaming one.

Second, blind the data at the beginning of the project. Remove names and other identifying features to put people at ease. In the beginning, everyone will like to think they are top performers, but in reality, their greatest fear is that they are in the bottom tail. After a while defenses come down as all realize they are most likely in the middle. Moreover, no one will be the highest performer on every measure. Nor will anyone consistently be the lowest. This means everyone has something to learn from someone and something to teach someone else.

When routinely examined, data variation can be harnessed to overcome resistance to change. Examining variation in outcomes, quality, or costs builds dissatisfaction with the current performance state because it is blatantly obvious that improvement is possible. It also provides a vision of what the future will look like—it is right there in the data. Finally, the discussions that happen when an organization becomes more data-focused help to identify achievable first steps in the transformation process.

Dissatisfaction * Vision * First Steps > Resistance

Successful transformation grows from shared agreement regarding the need for change, a clear vision, and achievable first steps. The achievable steps are only possible if there is sufficient capability. Shortfalls in any aspect of the formula create predictable reactions.

Formula of Change
Variation of the Gleicher's Formula

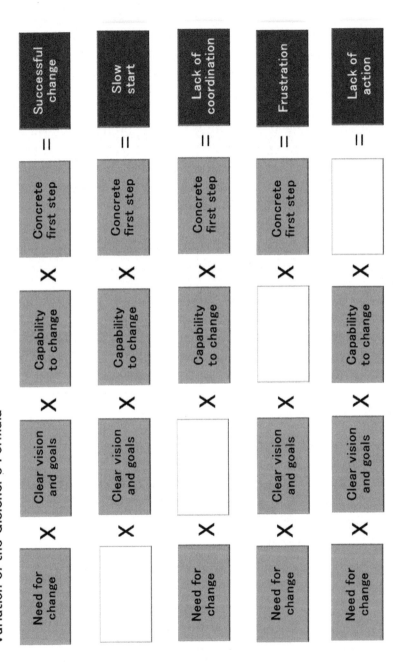

Need for change	X	Clear vision and goals	X	Capability to change	X	Concrete first step	=	Successful change
	X	Clear vision and goals	X	Capability to change	X	Concrete first step	=	Slow start
Need for change	X		X	Capability to change	X	Concrete first step	=	Lack of coordination
Need for change	X	Clear vision and goals	X		X	Concrete first step	=	Frustration
Need for change	X	Clear vision and goals	X	Capability to change	X		=	Lack of action

Dannemiller, K.D. & Jacobs, R.W. (1992) Changing the way organizations change. *The Journal of Applied Behavioral Science. 28(4) 480–498*

A lack of consensus regarding the need for change predictably leads to a slow start.

A murky vision or fuzzy goals will manifest as a lack of coordination. Lacking the capability to change produces frustration, while ambiguous first steps breed paralysis.

Variation in the delivery of healthcare has been observed for as long as, and wherever, anyone has looked. When seen through the eyes of manufacturing sciences it is indicative of inefficiency, waste, and harm—all of which can be true. The inefficiencies and waste in our current healthcare system are robbing our infrastructure and education system. The harm done by our current healthcare system is unconscionable. Action is required in order to build a healthcare system that creates better outcomes and provides excellent service for the dollars spent on it. But to recognize this and conclude that all variation should be eliminated is shortsighted. When seen through the eyes of an evolutionist, variation is a necessity that can identify beneficial adaptations. To paraphrase Charles Darwin: It is not the most intellectual that thrives; it is not the strongest that thrives; the one that thrives is the one best able to adapt and adjust to the changing environment in which it finds itself.

Variation does not need to be eliminated in healthcare; we have to learn from it and adapt.

Resources

»   Glover, J.A. (2008). The incidence of tonsillectomy in school children. *Proceedings of the Royal Society of Medicine*, 1938.31, 1219-36. Reprinted *Int J Epidemiol*, 37, 9-19.

»   Wennberg, J.E. (2010). *Tracking Medicine: A researcher's quest to understand healthcare*. Oxford: University Press.

»   Newhouse, J., & Graber, A. (Eds). (2013) *Variation in healthcare spending: Target decision making, not geography*. Washington, DC: Institute of Medicine.

»   Kotter, J. P. (2007). Leading change: Why transformation efforts fail. *Harvard Business Review*, 92, 107.

»   Dannemiller, K.D., & Jacobs, R.W. (1992) Changing the way organizations change. *The Journal of Applied Behavioral Science*, 28(4), 480-498.

»   Beckhard, R., Harris R.T. (1987) *Organizational Transitions* (2nd Ed). Reading, MA: Addison-Wesley Publishing.

CHAPTER 3

LOOKING FOR VALUE OPPORTUNITIES

Measurement is perhaps the most fundamental aspect of any transformation project. There are countless sayings in business along the lines of, "You can't manage what you can't measure." Not only do you need to track important metrics following a transformation, but you also must track these metrics prior to the implementation to understand whether the transformation is having the desired effect.

A colleague once relayed a story of one department struggling with some basic measurement issues. With all the advertisements and scholarly articles about "big data," enterprise-wide, cloud-based, data warehouse solutions, and the like it is easy to lose perspective. A substantial number of healthcare provider organizations still have difficulty calculating proportions. For example, it is common to hear of difficulties finding the proportion of patients with diabetes and an A1C level greater than nine who have not had an appointment in the past six months. My colleague's story revolved around a project meant to increase an obstetrics unit's volume of deliveries. The hospital leadership worked to increase the number of babies they delivered, but had no system for predicting how many babies they could expect to deliver during a given timeframe. Due to this lack of data, they routinely turned away pregnant mothers who were expected to deliver in a certain month out of concern that the hospital was going to be especially busy.

How did they know the month was going to be busy? And what does busy mean? Someone (usually the head of the department) had been documenting how many pregnant women were being seen by the clinic and their expected due dates. The department head then estimated how many of these mothers would actually deliver at their facility and how many deliveries the hospital could safely handle in a given period. The calculation went something like this: "250 mothers are expected to deliver in March, less 30 percent (due to various reasons: miscarriage, move out of town, etc.)." Therefore, the hospital would expect 175 mothers to deliver in March (250 x 70%). This projection was then compared to the department's capacity, which was defined as: "The hospital can safely handle 160 deliveries per month." When demand was expected to exceed capacity, no new patients with an expected delivery date in March were accepted. While the logic is sound, there are better and more robust methods to forecast these deliveries than by mere assumption.

Consequently, the hospital would routinely under-forecast deliveries and routinely miss their delivery targets.

Considerable time in healthcare is spent addressing such issues as predicting the volume of services several months in advance. And considerable money is spent advertising the quality of groups' services to in order to increase patient volume, and more time and money is then spent to improve capacity so as to meet the anticipated need. None of this effort and expense serves to increase the value of healthcare.

We measure many things in healthcare, but we do not measure value particularly well. In fact, most organizations do not measure value's fundamental building blocks. Value is the quotient derived from dividing the outcomes relevant to patients by the costs associated with achieving those outcomes. How can you begin measuring value? Start by understanding outcomes that matter to patients and then determine what it costs to achieve those outcomes. Remember, value increases when outcomes improve, or when outcomes remain steady but costs are reduced.

INSIGHTS AVAILABLE NOW

If you work in or run a hospital, you can find more than 200 publicly available data sets covering the performance of your healthcare organization. So even if you were not focused on the value your organization is creating, others have been. These data includes payment amounts reimbursed to the organization for care provided, the estimated costs to deliver the care, patients' perceptions of their experience within your organization, your rate of certain surgical procedures compared to state and national averages (or compared to your regional competitors), the proportion of your patients using hospice services during the last six months of their lives, the proportion of your patients being seen by ten or more doctors, and more.

Not every piece of data is available to every organization, but there are some data available on all but the smallest facilities, and these data are freely available. Yes, this material is a chore to retrieve, organize, and display, but the cost is small compared to the total amount spent on transformation efforts— to say nothing of the benefits reaped by studying the data. Furthermore, what you learn from the publicly available data can help inform and target your later efforts.

There is no need for an organization to invest in an enterprise-wide data infrastructure project if it uses the publicly available data to identify the medical conditions and care processes with the most room for improvement and savings, and then prioritizes efforts based on knowledge of local context.

Let me provide a fictitious example, keeping in mind that not every hospital makes available rates for every procedure. The figure below shows a comparison of procedures for four organizations plus the national average. The procedures are those that have been previously identified as opportunities for quick and substantial improvement in patient outcomes and reductions in cost.

Figure 3.1: Publicly Available Rates for Four Organizations

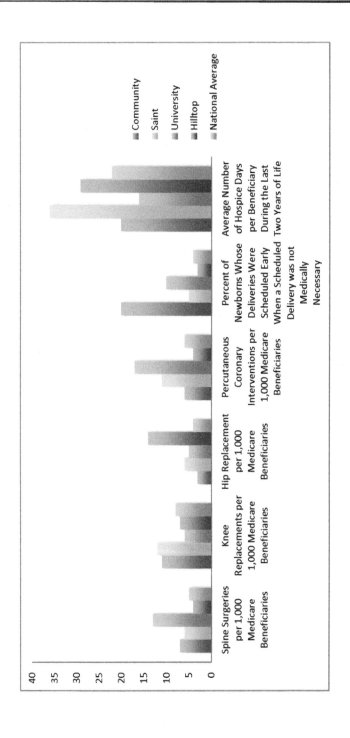

Imagine you are the chief executive of Community Hospital System. From publicly available sources, you have gathered data on your organization and your regional competitors: Saint Hospital, University Hospital, and Hilltop Regional. A careful review of the chart clearly shows your percentage of prematurely scheduled deliveries is four times the national average and double the nearest rival. Meanwhile, the number of hip replacements performed throughout your organizations was below the national average. Spine surgeries, knee replacements, percutaneous coronary interventions, and hospice use were near the national average. Your opportunity for quick and substantial improvement in patient outcomes, reductions in costs, and savings for payers lies in your process of care for women during pregnancy.

Let's now switch to Hilltop's perspective. Hilltop's rate of spine surgeries, knee replacements, percutaneous coronary interventions, and early elective inductions are already below the national average, and typically the lowest in the region. Plus, Hilltop's average number of hospice days per Medicare beneficiary is higher than the national average. Meanwhile, Hilltop's rate of hip replacements is twice as high as any of its competitors and nearly three times the national average.

From a policy standpoint, it appears Hilltop's rate of hip replacements could be wasteful. There is little reason to believe the patients in the region have hips that are more arthritic than would typically be found across the country, especially when their spines and knees do not seem to require so much intervention. Hilltop would be wise to start transformation efforts with a focus on how they care for patients with degenerative arthritis of the hip.

Data are publicly available for many more medical conditions and processes, and they can be gathered to compare your organization's utilization rates, patients' assessment of their care experience, estimated costs, and reimbursements against state and national averages, regional competitors, US News & World Report's top performing hospitals, or the flagship facility for accountable care organizations that successfully earned savings. Organizing the data as described above will turn the raw data into insightful information that will help start or better focus your transformation efforts.

External data sources can help an organization know where to start, but transformation requires change from within. The next section of this chapter highlights what it takes to begin collecting, retrieving, organizing, and displaying data from within an organization with a focus on measures necessary for tracking and improving the value of care delivered.

INTERNAL DATA

WHAT

What to measure requires special consideration. Many times in healthcare, we default to an existing or easily available measure that does not really capture the intent of our efforts. Does your chosen measure matter to patients? Have you asked to be certain? Increasing the value of the healthcare we deliver calls for us to improve the outcomes that matter to patients and/or decrease the costs associated with achieving those outcomes. Measures such as A1C or FEV1 or even blood pressure provide usual information to us as clinicians, but they do not represent outcomes that matter to patients.

Determining what to measure can be tricky. It helps to look at existing literature to make sure you are considering the strengths and the weaknesses of your selected data points. You want a pragmatic list of meaningful measures because there is a cost for reporting, retrieving, organizing, and displaying each variable you select. Choose your measures with great care.

You will probably want at least one outcome measure that matters to patients and some measure of the cost of the care provided to produce the outcome.

WHERE

Where do your data live now, if they are already collected or reported? Where will you store them if you will be collecting them yourself? Different data points live in different locations. Some live in the medical record, some in a condition-specific registry, and others in the billing or appointment system. Still more are available through online resources that monitor physician, clinic, hospital, and regional performance. Retrieving data from multiple sources and linking each source to a specific patient or group of patients can be tricky and often requires the assistance of a data engineer. Many projects will require pulling data from the same systems regardless of the project. For example, the need for data from the medical record, billing, and appointment systems are very common. The first few times the data engineer attempts to retrieve and organize the data, the effort can be clumsy and take a long time. This is why is helpful for an organization to have a data engineer working to support improvement and transformation efforts. Over time, as the engineer shares what she has learned, it becomes easier to automate the retrieval, organization, and display of common data points.

WHO

Who will retrieve, organize, and display the data? It may be a single person or it may be two or three. Was this person or team involved in planning the project implementation? Whoever it is, they need to be part of the scoping and diagnostic phases of each project. Many well-intentioned projects begin by defining the what, where, and when of a measure that matters to patients and costs, but then fall apart when the only thought about "who" is "Oh, we can have the receptionist or nurse hand that survey to patients and get it back as the patient leaves," or, "We'll have the patients do that online and our nurse can check it for errors near the end of his day," or, "Let's just run the cost report we've always used."

WHEN

When will the data be retrieved, organized, and displayed? Data that are as close to real time as possible have the most influence on processes. Displays based on data that are months or even years removed from the process have little influence. In fact, providing feedback with data that are old, and where the means to influence the data are unclear, breeds cynicism and resentment.

A critical part of improvement and transformation work is to make routine the retrieval, organization, and display of measures that matter to patients and drive value.

Now we will look at essential information regarding outcomes that matter to patients and costs.

CHAPTER 4

HOW TO MEASURE VALUE

R emember, value increases when outcomes improve, and value also increases when outcomes remain steady, but costs are lowered. How can you begin measuring value? Start by understanding outcomes that matter to patients and then understanding what it costs to achieve those outcomes.

OUTCOMES THAT MATTER TO PATIENTS

We need to know what matters most to patients, and we need to stop assuming we know. Surgical oncologists assume that 71% of their patients with breast cancer believe "saving their breast" is a top priority, but just 17% of patients with breast cancer rate "saving my breast" as a top priority (Lee, et. al, 2010). In Ontario, Canada, researchers gave imaging studies and medical records of patients with knee arthritis to orthopedic surgeons and asked them to identify patients eligible for knee replacement surgery. The researchers then went to those patients and asked about their willingness to undergo the procedure. Fifteen percent of the patients deemed eligible were interested (Hawker et al., 2001).

When asked, patients tell us pain matters to them. The less, the better, but it's not the only thing that matters. Their ability to fulfill the roles they perceive for themselves also matters. A sense of well-being matters, as does perceived health status. Regardless of the medical diagnosis, a patient is not doing well if he tells you he feels unwell and things are getting worse.

Patients also care whether their healthcare providers know them personally. Nobody wants to be thought of only as a diagnosis. Patients also care whether the members of their healthcare team work together well. It is distressing for patients when one provider does not know what another provider has done or plans to do.

Of all of the aforementioned priorities, pain levels are the only routinely measured variable today, so unless you are taking explicit steps to find out what matters most to your patients, you are likely to be missing important information.

How will you measure outcomes that matter to patients? Is there a reliable, valid, and widely accepted method for measuring an outcome that is meaningful to patients? While many healthcare organizations have mission statements declaring their commitment to patient-centered care, the truth is many providers and administrators have no idea how to measure it, nor do they know the difference between patient-centered, patient-reported, and/ or patient-generated data.

Patient-centered outcomes matter to patients. We know this from interviews and focus groups with thousands of patients, and from commonsense. Survival is a patient-centered outcome. Readmission rates are patient-centered. As mentioned earlier, other common healthcare measures, such as blood pressure, forced expiratory volume, and even radiographic evidence of boney fusion following spine surgery, are not patient-centered. Immediately following spinal fusion surgery, outcomes that are patient-centered include pain, and the ability to perform daily activities such as getting out of bed, showering, and using the toilet. In the longer term, pain still matters and so does the ability to perform the tasks that distinguish the different roles a person assumes at home, at work and in his or her community.

Patients, not healthcare providers, supply **patient-reported outcomes** (PROs). Similar to satisfaction questionnaires, PROs are surveys, but instead of asking about the visit, the patients are asked about their perceptions of their health. Shocking to no one but healthcare providers and perhaps researchers, these surveys provide tremendous insight into what patients value most about their health. Patient-reported outcomes grew out of the Medical Outcomes Studies (MOS) from the 1990s that asked patients hundreds of questions about their health, their sense of well-being, and their ability to complete their daily activities in the roles they defined for themselves. Over time, researchers categorized the questions into eight dimensions that included physical, mental, and social health. The researchers were eventually able to cull the list of questions to a few dozen meant to be applicable to all adults, regardless of their medical diagnosis. Broad surveys like these that are suitable for use regardless of a patient's diagnosis are considered generic surveys for this reason.

Other researchers created patient-reported surveys for specific medical conditions. Condition-specific, patient-reported health surveys are now available for many conditions, including back pain, knee pain, colitis and migraines. Condition-specific surveys were created because researchers recognized that a patient might seek help for his knee pain and stiffness, and receive treatments that decrease the pain and improve his function, all the while reporting his general health to be normal and fine. That is, the generic survey would not be able to detect the original difficulty or a change in health status. At the same time, a condition-specific survey for knee pain, by targeting only the knee, could theoretically miss important perceptions a patient may have regarding how the knee pain affects his physical and mental well-being. Because generic and condition-specific measures each had strengths and weaknesses, most experts suggested using both.

Both generic and condition-specific surveys are becoming more widespread because of their importance in understanding value in healthcare. Theoretically, it would be possible to calculate the value of healthcare for a patient by dividing the change in a measureable outcome, (e.g., health status as reported by the patient) by the cost of providing the goods and services that led to the outcome.

Patient-generated outcomes are co-created by scientists working closely with patients to ensure the outcome matters to patients, is reported by patients, and is collected in a manner that makes sense to patients. As such, they are state of the art for understanding what outcomes matter most to patients.

There has been an eruption of patient-reported surveys purporting to be patient-centered, but when examined carefully, they are homegrown and lack a rigorous assessment of their reliability and validity. The only acceptable reason to use a survey instrument without solid documentation of its psychometric properties is if you are building a new one. When deciding how you will measure the impact of your improvement efforts, keep in mind the path to creating a reliable and valid patient-generated assessment of health status is several years long and requires a scientist with training specific for the task (a psychometrician).

Even a clinician who is knowledgeable about patient-reported measures is likely to have a limited view of their usefulness. The view is confined to outcome reporting, where patients' scores are aggregated and the data are fed back to the clinician quarterly. There is a lot to be learned with this approach, but the feedback it supplies arrives months later. Remote feedback like this is similar to having a 30-second delay between twisting the hot water knob in a shower and the change in water temperature. It is frustrating and impossible to get comfortable. Most clinicians do not know that in addition to the aggregated feedback mechanism, it is possible to feedforward data in a manner that supports clinical decisions in real time at the point of care, providing actionable information that can be used to create greater value. These data can then be used to support patient intake, triage, and navigation along a care pathway. It helps to switch from thinking about patient-reported *outcomes* (PROs) to thinking about patient-reported health status measures (HSMs).

Technology allows for the collection of HSMs via patient portals or using apps before the clinical encounter. The data can be organized and displayed in a manner that improves the patient intake process by providing the clinic staff with information regarding the patient's current status and trends if it is a follow-up visit. The staff can also use this information to triage patients to the appropriate care provider at the appropriate time and to inform the patient's navigation through a care pathway over time.

The figure below shows a pre-appointment HSM. The red arrow farthest to the right highlights the patient-reported functional status. It is easy to identify the activities that are proving difficult. The second red arrow shows the gap between the age- and gender-adjusted normal values, represented by the dotted line, across the eight domains of health assessed by the SF-36.

FIGURE 4.1: PATIENT 1'S REPORTED HEALTH STATUS MEASURE DISPLAYED PRIOR TO CLINICAL ENCOUNTER

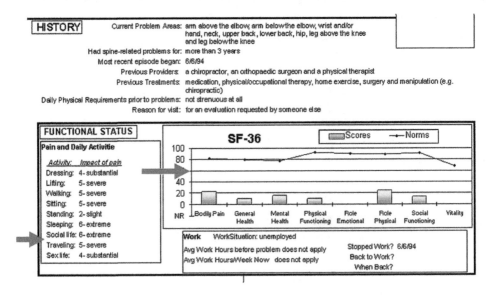

A quick glance reveals a patient reporting diminished health status, including a sense of physical and mental well-being as well as an ability to function physically and to fulfill the emotional and physical roles as the patient sees them. When HSMs become part of routine clinical practice in this manner, they become as informative as imaging studies. Below is the magnetic resonance image for the same patient.

FIGURE 4.2: PATIENT 1'S MRI

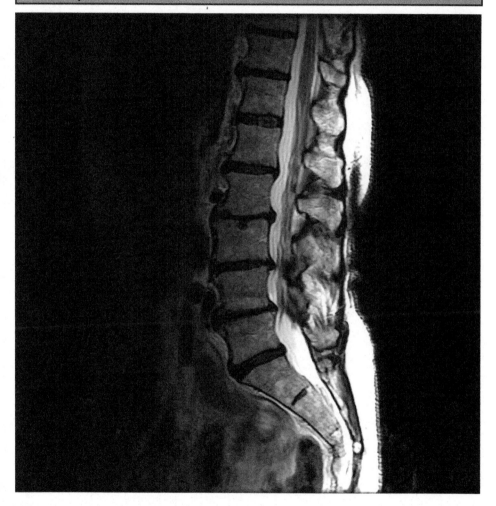

The MRI reveals age-related changes, and different specialists may argue over the efficacy of any single treatment approach, be it exercise, injections, or surgery. Couple the MRI with the HSM, however, and we provide information that reveals single form of care is likely to substantially improve the patient's health. A multidisciplinary approach is likely best to address his functional limitations and physical, emotional, and mental health. Furthermore, reviewing the HSM results with the patient can help to clarify and enlighten the clinician's understanding of what matters most to the patient and to help them collaborate in order to find the best next step.

A second case reinforces how the use of HSMs provides clinicians with actionable information at the point of service, in much the same way as an MRI, and together they further enhance each other. Let's begin with the imaging study.

FIGURE 4.3: PATIENT 2'S MRI

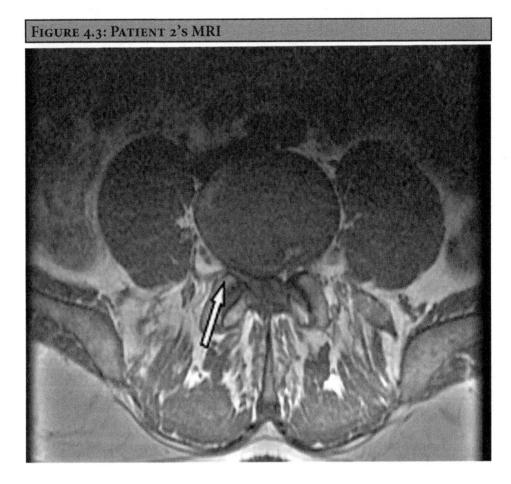

This is an image of the patient laying on her back undergoing a magnetic resonance image (MRI) of her spine. This image shows her kidneys on each side of a spinal disc directly in the center. The white arrow points to a tear in the disk with a substantial herniation of material beyond its normal confines. This is a common image seen in patients before an operation to repair/remove the herniation. The patient's HSMs, however, suggest a different story.

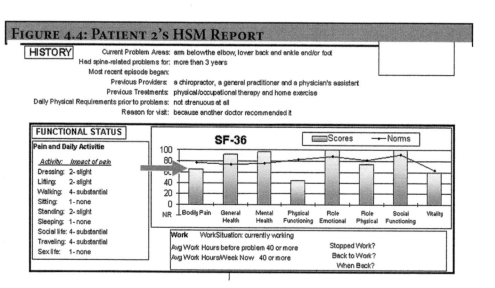

FIGURE 4.4: PATIENT 2'S HSM REPORT

Here the red arrow shows a dotted line representing normal values for women of the same age. In this example, the patient's current state is near or above the normal for almost every measure. It would be difficult for surgery to improve the patient's situation further.

A final example reinforces the value of HSMs. In the figure below you can see the patient is reporting her greatest difficulty with her mental health and her ability to fulfill the emotional roles she defines for herself. She is also having extreme difficulty sleeping.

FIGURE 4.5: PATIENT 3'S HSM REPORT

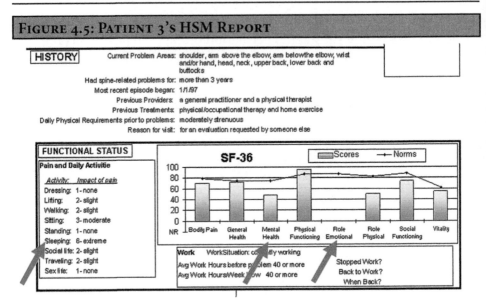

In the following MRI image the patient is in an upright position, facing to the left. The MRI slice is of her lower back/lumbar region. The most easily observed detail is the thin disk near the bottom of the spine. But more important is a fragmented piece of disk lying out of position, behind the bony vertebra and narrowing space for the nearby nerve, as indicated by the white arrow. This is also a common image among patients receiving a recommendation for spine surgery.

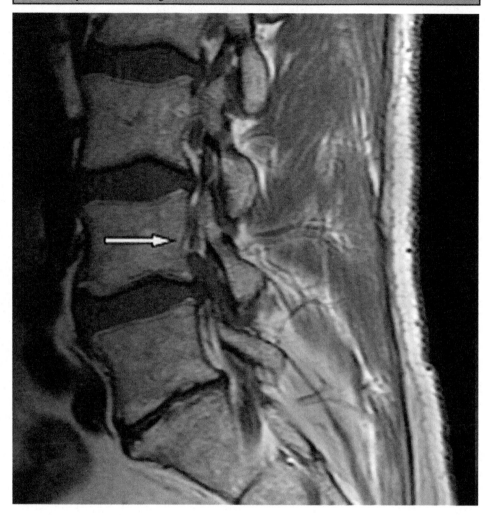

At this point, a conversation is needed between Patient 3 and her surgeon. Surgery for a disk herniation can help relieve pain, especially pain from a pinched nerve. Surgery for a disk herniation is likely to have much less effect on a patient's mental well-being, unless the diminished capacity and sleep difficulties can be directly linked to the physical ailment. A collaborative conversation between the patient and surgeon can make sure they are on the same page regarding options, risks, benefits, expectations, and what matters most to the patient. Furthermore, when patient and provider understanding is high and confusion is low, the entire practice staff benefits from the clarity of purpose. Non-emergent calls decline, missed or duplicate orders are reduced, and return appointments are kept open for patients needing additional action, not clarifying miscommunication.

These three clinical examples illustrate how HSMs, used at the point of service, and within the clinical exchange between patient and provider, can help improve communication and inform key leverage points for enhancing the value of care, patient intake, triage, and navigation.

Costs

Understanding value requires knowledge of costs. How will you measure costs? The terms can be confusing because perspective matters. For example, what it costs a hospital to deliver healthcare is not the same as what Medicare spends to pay for the treatment of Medicare beneficiaries, but the amount Medicare spends on healthcare is a large portion of the cost of healthcare for our country.

To develop a shared language among those of us transforming the delivery of care, we'll take the hospital or provider's perspective. From this standpoint, costs are the expenses paid in order to deliver care. These include salaries for the doctors, nurses and therapists, and the supplies they need to directly provide care to patients, as well as the indirect costs of paying administrators, maintaining infrastructure and educating trainees. Some of the direct and indirect costs remain fixed regardless of the volume of patients receiving care, while others vary depending on the number of patients flowing through the system.

Charges are billed to payers for each procedure performed and each supply used to care for a patient. In healthcare, each hospital negotiates with each payer to establish a discounted price. The hospitals and payers have traditionally guarded the discount amount in an attempt to leverage the best possible deal. Very large hospital systems and prestigious institutions in regions with a small number of insurance organizations can offer very small discounts. Smaller and less prestigious organizations, especially in regions containing several different payer options, have to offer large discounts or risk being dropped from the payers' list of providers. It's important to remain on each payer's list, because dropping off the list means patients covered by the payer would have to pay the charged amount in full and the hospital would lose business.

The government-run payer systems, Medicare and Medicaid, are so large they can set their own reimbursement rates. Because of this market power, the government payers' rates are below the prices charged by the hospital. There are two ways to look at this gap between government payers and listed prices. In the traditional, hospital-centric view, the gap signals an underpayment for services that have to be filled by raising the prices charged to other payers. Hospital administrators call this cost shifting. Alternatively, it is possible to view the gap between government payers and listed prices as a signal of a hospital's market power and negotiating skill. A prestigious facility, or one without much competition, has the ability to set higher prices than a less-prestigious hospital or one in a flooded market. The hospital's market power allows it to set higher prices, which, in turn, creates an illusion of more severe underpayment from Medicare and Medicaid.

The disagreement over cost shifting illustrates how little we know about costs, charges, and reimbursements in healthcare. Understanding charges and their relationship to true costs has become a priority for healthcare administrators, researchers, and policy makers. The latter would like to contain the rate of growth in the amount our nation spends on healthcare. They are concerned that ballooning healthcare expenditures due to an aging population will require higher taxes and less investment in other societal priorities such as education and infrastructure. However, slowing the growth in national healthcare spending creates a sense of scarcity for healthcare administrators. They understand that in a less expansive environment, institutions will need to reign in their costs of producing healthcare services, and they fear their current knowledge of their organization's costs is not adequate for the negotiations that take place with payers. For this reason, knowledge of an organization's costs is not only a competitive advantage—it is a necessity for maintaining operating margins.

Techniques for allocating costs range from the generic to the specific. There is no consensus among industry experts regarding the best method. The desired outcome, regardless of allocation method, is to assign institutional costs to the patients that created the need for them. It becomes obvious, when attempting to do so, that some costs are directly due to activities involved in patient care and some costs belong to the institution as a whole. Direct costs are clearly associated with patient care. Everything else is an indirect cost.

Allocating indirect costs makes cost allocation in healthcare either exciting or painful to establish, depending on your disposition. What follows are several methods for allocation of costs and their various issues and benefits.

The **direct method of allocating indirect costs** allocates non-revenue activities to revenue-producing activities. This is a relatively simple method but can be distorted by the fact that some non-revenue activities provide services to other non-revenue units. For example, the housekeeping service cleans administrative offices but neither housekeeping nor administration produce revenue in the healthcare industry. The **reciprocal method** acknowledges this interdependency, but is more complex. The complex allocation can also make decision-making more difficult because revenue centers are assigned costs, but managers within the revenue centers have no ability to manage those assigned costs. The **step-down method** attempts to bridge the simplicity of the direct method and the complexity of the reciprocal by allowing non-revenue producing departments to allocate costs to each other. But, the step-down method requires a sequential allocation process AND the order used to enter costs will affect the outcome, making it somewhat less trusted.

The **ratio of cost-to-charge (RCC) method** involves allocating direct and indirect costs of care based on the amount charged to the payer. For example, the costs of housekeeping and administration would be considered twice as high for a patient undergoing a $20,000 procedure compared to a patient having a $10,000 procedure. This is simple, and easy to perform and understand, yet there are obvious limitations—the true administrative costs associated with a $20,000 procedure are not likely to be 1,000% greater than a $200 office visit.

The **relative value unit (RVU) method** is considered more accurate than the RCC because it incorporates clinical acuity. Development of RVU values requires clinical expertise, collaboration across departments, and considerable time for revision as diagnostic codes are added, subtracted and modified across the industry.

All allocation methods become messy as they attempt to disseminate shared costs like administration or housekeeping across all units served. The imprecise nature of the process is inherently unsatisfying to academics and policy makers. Nevertheless, administrators want the best available data to inform their decisions and to help them maintain operating margins. The greater accuracy possible from more advanced techniques must be weighed against the additional costs of collecting and analyzing the necessary data. In addition, an allocation method should be chosen not only based on its accuracy and ease of use, but also its ability to provide timely and actionable information to decision makers.

Activity-based costing (ABC) is an allocation method employing a variation of the step-down method to deal with indirect costs. First described by Kaplan, it was created to provide actionable information by identifying the activities required to deliver healthcare services to a particular group of patients or a particular service line. In the ABC view, resources such as salaries and materials are "consumed" by the activities required to deliver healthcare. A cost object—typically a patient, a service line, or department—consumes the activities. Any activity that incurs costs is considered a cost-driver.

Shortly after it was developed, healthcare administrators saw great potential for ABC because of the ability to assess costs at smaller units of analysis, potentially down to the individual patient level, which might provide better information and enable better decision-making. Yet, in practice, the ABC's data requirements and resultant analytic burden proved very large. This burden outweighed the advantages of somewhat greater relevance and accuracy.

Each allocation method described contains some arbitrary choices. In the past, the limitations associated with each method have been obscured by the continued growth of the healthcare industry. Precise knowledge of costs was not necessary because reimbursements always went up. However, now that the growth in healthcare reimbursements has slowed, the limitations of the methods for understanding costs have become more problematic. Healthcare scientists, policy makers, and administrators are now focused on finding a method that best informs operational decision-making in a timely manner and in a resource-constrained environment.

The quest for a highly accurate, actionable, yet low-intensity method capable of informing institutional decision makers led Kaplan and colleagues at Harvard to devise time-driven, activity-based costing (TDABC). The authors suggest TDABC was a substantial breakthrough in the field of cost allocation, but no empirical data currently exist to either confirm or refute this assertion.

The goal is to strive for a balance of information useful for decision-making without requiring onerous data collection or uninformed estimations (guessing), but appropriately allocating indirect costs remains problematic. The evaluation of time estimates can also be problematic in TDABC models. The team can estimate the time (also called standard times), or time can be measured by an observer (actual times). The differences between the two can be substantial, and leadership may be reluctant to accept estimations. However, direct observation will alter the behavior of the observed and can create distrust and unease. For these reasons, creating time equations should be an iterative process and conducted with a spirit of inquiry, not judgment.

Increasing the complexity of the process map, the unit cost estimation, and the time equations are all possible. Accuracy may improve through additional complexity but at the cost of an increased data collection and analysis burden, not to mention the costs of the working group spending time on mapping and modeling instead of caring for patients.

No allocation method is perfect. The objective is to be "good enough" for decision-making without imposing additional costs or an undue data collection and analytic burden. The process maps and cost calculations should be as simple as possible.

To assess the sustainability of any process improvement effort, changes to institutional costs must be compared to reimbursement levels. An organization seeking to meet targeted reductions in reimbursements, as required by shared-savings arrangements in an accountable care organization, for example, will need to compare changes to both institutional costs and reimbursement levels in order to maintain an operating margin.

To blunt any potential financial losses stemming from limitations inherent with measuring cost, the deployment of any new allocation method, such as TDABC, should take place first in pilot locations. Once a process is mapped out, it is relatively easy to update and expand any relevant calculations. The most significant savings come from questions regarding location and personnel. First ask, "Is there a better or less expensive location for this process?" Second, ask, "Are we using all personnel to the top of their license?" Many times a better, less expensive location can be found and less expensive, but highly trained care providers can meet the needs of most patients. In addition, many processes can be improved by removing accumulated waste. Like items in a drawer, clutter happens to processes that are left unattended. Removing duplicate and unused items leads to less wasted time trying to find needed items. Removing the waste improves efficiency.

Before committing considerable resources to developing expansive process maps and TDABC models, consider that process improvement efforts have not reliably produced the predicted savings in societal expenses or institutional costs. Time-driven, activity-based costing may have potential to help achieve institutional cost savings while organizations attempt to meet decreasing reimbursement goals as part of an accountable care agreement, but TDABC has not been rigorously examined in academic literature. Anecdotal reports of successful cost reduction using the method in one location have not generalized to other sites.

Consider instead the idea of building an organization's capacity for self-awareness about value. Most organizations today do not understand their costs. Most do not measure outcomes that matter to patients. Without awareness of costs and outcomes, they cannot assess the value of the healthcare they deliver.

The healthcare industry seems to be a chaotic place due to new legislation and the transformation from volume-based to value-based payment models. But it is important for our country's sake that we continue to slow the growth rate in our national expenditure on healthcare. It is also true that a decreasing growth rate in the country's healthcare expenditures presents a threat to any particular institution because the country's saved expenditures are the institution's lost revenue. This conflict is the heart of the problem faced by those working to reform healthcare delivery. Slowing the growth rate is good for our country and cities, and it is survivable by our healthcare-providing institutions, even if not as profitable as in the past, if leaders build the systems and procedures necessary to understand their patients' outcomes and the cost of the care required to achieve those outcomes.

Resources

»   Lee, C.N., Dominik R., Levin, C.A., Barry, M.J., Cosenza, C., O'Connor, A.M., Mulley, A.G. Jr., & Sepucha, K.R. (2010). Development of instruments to measure the quality of breast cancer treatment decisions. *Health Expectations*, 13(3), 258–72. doi:10.1111/j.1369-7625.2010.00600.x

»   Hawker, G.A., Wright, J.G., Coyte P.C., Williams, J.I., Harvey, B., Glazier, R., Wilkins, A., & Badley, E.M. (2001). Determining the need for hip and knee arthroplasty: the role of clinical severity and patients' preferences. *Medical Care*, 39(3), 206–16.

»   Stewart, A.L., & Ware, J.E. (Eds). (1992) *Measuring functioning and well-being: The Medical Outcomes Study Approach*. Durham, NC: Duke University Press.

»   Ware, J.E., & Sherbourne, C.D. (1992). The MOS 36-item short-form health survey (SF-36): I. Conceptual framework and item selection. *Medical Care*, 30, 473-483.

»   Walsh T., Hanscom B., Lurie J.D., & Weinstein J.N. (2003). Is a condition-specific instrument for patients with low back pain/leg symptoms really necessary? The responsiveness of the Oswestry Disability Index, MODEMS, and the SF-36. *Spine* 15(28m), 6, 607-615.

»   The Center for Medicare & Medicaid Innovation. *Priority measures for monitoring and evaluation.* http://innovation.cms.gov/Files/x/PriorityMsrMontEval.pdf

»   Stensland, J., Gaumer Z.R., & Miller M.E. (2010) Private-payer profits can induce negative Medicare margins. *Health Affairs* 2010. 29(5),1045-1051.

»   Frakt, A. (2014) The end of hospital cost shifting and the quest for hospital productivity. *Health Services Research*. 49(1), 1-10.

»   Carey, R.G., & Lloyd, R.C. (2001) *Measuring Quality Improvement in Healthcare – A guide to statistical process control applications*. Milwaukee, WI: Quality Press.

»   Berwick, W., R. Matthews, & Scanlon, C. (2010). *Achieving clinical and operational excellence: how to establish healthcare service line costs*. Redwood Shores, CA: Oracle Corp.

»   Weinstein, J.N., Brown, P.W., Hanscom, B., Walsh ,T., & Nelson, E. (2000). Designing an ambulatory clinical practice for outcomes improvement: From vision to reality, The Spine Center at Dartmouth-Hitchcock, year one. *Quality Management Health Care.* 8(2), 1-20.

» Holdren, J.P. & Lander, E.S. (Co-Chairs). (May 2014) *Better health care and lower costs: Accelerating improvement through systems engineering.* President's Council of Advisors on Science and Technology.

» Finkler, S., Ward, D., & Baker, J. (2007), *Essentials of Cost Accounting for Healthcare Organizations,* 3rd ed. Sudbury, Massachusetts: Jones and Bartlett.

» Gapenski, L., (2011) *Healthcare Finance: An introduction to accounting and financial management.* 4th ed., Chicago, IL: Health Administration Press.

» Kaplan, R.S. (May 2014). Introduction to Time-Driven Activity-Based Costing in Healthcare. Presented in Dublin, Ireland. http://hse.ie/eng/services/news/newsfeatures/masterclass/programme/CostMeasurement.pdf

» Kaplan, R. & Porter, M. (2011) How to solve the cost crisis in health care. *Harvard Business Review.*

» Black, N. (2013). Patient reported outcome measures could help transform healthcare. *BMJ.* 346:f167

» Cady, S.H., Jacobs, J., Koller, R., & Spalding, J. (2014). The Change Formula. *OD Practitioner.* 46(3), 32-39.

» Gervais, M., Levant, Y. & Ducrocq, C. (2010). *Time-Driven Activity-Based Costing: an initial appraisal through a longitudinal case study. JAMAR.* 8(2), 1-20.

» Higgins, A., et al. (2011). Early lessons from Accountable Care Models in the private sector: Partnerships between health plans and providers. *Health Affairs,* 2011. 30(9), 1718-1727.

» Nelson, L., (2012). *Lessons from Medicare's Demonstration Projects on Disease Management, Care Coordination, and Value-Based Payment.* Washington, DC: Congressional Budget Office.

» Reinhardt, U. (2012) Divid et impera: Protecting the growth of health care incomes (costs). *Health Econ.* 21, 41-54.

CHAPTER 5

THE SIGNIFICANCE OF MICROSYSTEMS

One item on our Spine Center patient dashboards stuck out more than others—the mental component summary score, or MCS. The MCS was a composite score built from all eight domains of health assessed by the SF-36, but most heavily weighted to the mental health, vitality, and mental role questions.

The component summary scores are normalized so that a score of 50 is considered a normal score, and 95% of the population should score between 30 and 70. This also meant just 2.5% of a population should score below 30 or above 70. A low MCS score for someone visibly stressed because of, or in addition to, their back pain was not surprising, but some eyebrows were raised by just how low these scores were for so many of our patients. Not only were the low scores very low, we seldom witnessed a score above 55. We were also surprised by the number of patients who appeared "normal" during our verbal interactions, but who reported their mental well-being to be far below expected values for a person of similar age and gender in their self-reported surveys. Just how different was our sample of patients compared to a normally distributed population? Well, instead of the expected 2.5% with scores below 30, our sample reported just over 14%, with scores more than two standard deviations below the population mean.

To explore these surprises further, I started to make it a habit to thank my patients for completing the survey and then use the results to drive my interactions with them. This was awkward for me at first. I was accustomed to asking a sequence of questions that were predetermined by the form we used to help guide our medical notes. I worked hard to make my interactions feel natural while completing the form, by mentally keeping tally, jotting down quick notes, or sometimes typing on my computer while my patients spoke.

Interestingly, I realized that my patients seemed happiest with our interactions when I wrote down or entered some data while we talked. They were unhappy if I typed away as though dictating their comments, because it seemed as though I was not paying sufficient attention to them. However, it also was worrying to them if I did not write anything down because I was creating the impression that I did not care enough to take note of important things.

After years of following this same pattern for taking a history, I now had new data to incorporate, but it was awkward. Initially, I looked over the data outside the exam room, and then entered and conducted the interview and exam in my usual manner. This led to quizzical looks from patients as they asked why they had filled out the survey in the waiting room. I'd point to the survey and say, "The results are right here." This would typically be followed up by, "How did I do?" as if the survey was a test.

Over time, I found a solution to this issue that consisted of briefly reviewing the data outside the exam room, introducing myself to the patient as I entered the room, and then showing them the printed data and thanking them for completing the survey. I explained that it helped me to understand them and to treat them better. I would then ask for their help in understanding their answers.

A typical scenario would consist of me showing the form to a patient and explaining the normal or expected values, pointing to various points that were below average and asking them to tell me more about the ways in which their spine pains affected various aspects of their well-being. In this manner, a low physical-functioning score would lead to a discussion regarding what, specifically, they could not do as well as they needed or wanted. Similarly, a low MCS score served as an easy launching point for a discussing how their mood had been while dealing with their pain.

Using the data in this way took some getting used to, but after a few weeks I came to appreciate the quick insights it provided. I also grew accustomed to incorporating the new information into the old forms that were still required for administrative purposes.

Not everyone came to appreciate the new information in the same way. Some of my colleagues did not acknowledge the data with their patients, or even in their record of the visit. They simply continued doing what they had always done. This issue led us to creating a system that would automatically upload the data to the medical record.

At first, I wondered whether the recalcitrant physicians were seeing the same patterns that I saw, so I asked. There did not seem to be much of a difference, but there was reason to suspect that orthopedic surgeons, neurologists, and anesthesiologists would be seeing patients with different profiles from those seen by primary care providers or physical therapists.

The beautiful thing was, we could look. If all providers saw similar patients, it was not difficult to gather de-identified scores for a week or a month, code them by provider type, and do statistical tests to see if the observed values were different from the expected values. We did this several times and each time we found no substantial difference in pain or function scores across our multiple provider types. We did, however, notice one large difference between some providers, but it was not associated with provider type. In fact, we could find nothing in our data that could explain the difference.

Our data revealed substantial variation in the rate at which some providers referred patients with low MCS scores to behavioral medicine specialists. Some providers referred almost all of their patients with MCS scores below 30 to see one of our specialists. It was easy to do. Our multidisciplinary clinic had psychologists and social workers in adjacent offices. Despite the proximity, however, other providers never referred patients with low MCS scores to these trained behavioral medicine specialists.

One interpretation was to assume the high referral rates were among primary care or other holistic provider types, and the low referral rates were among highly specialized surgeons. That assumption was false. Provider training did not explain the variation.

We launched an education campaign that included displaying the variation in referral rates and detailing the evidence supporting the use of behavioral medicine for the treatment of anxiety and depression—the two most common mood disturbances associated with a low MCS score. The education campaign helped, but only a little. The overall rate of referral rose slightly and the range from highest to lowest rate narrowed enough to notice, but nowhere near to where we had hoped. Given the strength of the evidence supporting the integration of behavioral medicine into care plans for patients with mood disorders, something more was needed.

Our first action was to better understand our measure. We considered external data sources for comparison, but at that time there were no other facilities using the MCS score as an intake measure, rather than an outcome measure.

Our second action was taken to settle a disagreement. Some providers felt that every patient with an MCS score of 30 or less should be referred to one of our behavioral specialists. Others, however, felt that score was too low and some patients with higher scores and needing help could miss an effective treatment. Still others countered that our behavioral specialist staff could be inundated with patients not needing the care if the score was set too high. In a perverse way, too high of a cutoff score could make it more difficult for patients with the most need to get a timely appointment.

We needed to determine the appropriate score for a referral decision with some precision in order to settle the disagreement. To do so, we imbedded anxiety and depression condition-specific surveys into the patient-reported measures we gathered. As described earlier, condition-specific measures are generally better than generic measures at determining small, yet meaningful, differences in the condition of interest. In a few months, we had the data we needed from several hundred patients.

We then used statistical techniques to compare the results from the patients' condition-specific scores for depression and anxiety with their MCS scores from the generic SF-36 survey. Our analysis found that an MCS score of slightly less than 35 provided the best balance between a score that was so low it would miss patients who needed help and one that was too high and clogged our system with patients who did not need the care.

This result helped settle an argument among academics, but it did not change the variation in our referral rates to behavioral medicine for patients self-reporting mental and emotional distress. The process of care our system had adapted continued to churn almost as if it was immune to new information. Data alone was not sufficient to alter our care process.

Ultimately, we realized we needed to understand our current process of care from our patients' perspective. We asked for their help, and they were happy to contribute. We explained our desire to understand the process of care they received. We provided the patients with a clipboard, a pencil and a paper form with three columns. The first column was for noting their location in the office/practice, the second for their activity and the people (our staff) they interacted with, and the third for the time in each location or for each interaction. The first row was mundane. A typical entry read, "waiting room", "waiting/just me", "8:52 a.m." However, a more interesting story followed. Subsequent entries read, "moved to doctor's room", "just me", "8:54 a.m." Then, "In doctor's room", "nurse asked about medications", "9-9:05 a.m." And the next, "Doctor arrives 9:10", "She says I need to see a PT." "PT arrives 9:30" etc.

We then used the data from patients to map the processes of our care. The process maps were shocking for the time patients spent alone or performing redundant tasks that added no value to their care. We became inspired to remove this waste. More importantly, the action we needed to take to improve our referral rates to behavioral medicine for patients with self-reported emotional distress, as signaled by an MCS score of 35 or less, was jumping off those maps.

The maps differed for every provider. The maps also told us that every patient interacted with at least four of us, from the check-in receptionist, to an assistant, and then the provider, and then our check-out receptionist. We considered this collection of our staff plus the patient and the data about the patient a **microsystem**.

Most microsystems recognized the patient's MCS score only after the provider had entered the exam room and began talking with the patient. Some providers asked patients about their moods and mental health. A few shared the MCS score with patients, using it as a conversation starter. These two approaches were likely to lead to a referral to behavioral medicine, but the rates were still less than 60%.

A few providers had referral rates over 90%. How? They achieved this by reconfiguring their microsystem.

It turned out the providers with a high referral rate were not actually making the referral. Instead, they asked the clinic assistants to check the patient's MCS score as they escorted the patient to the clinical exam room. If the MCS score was less than 35, the assistant was instructed to page the behavioral medicine specialist right away—*before the provider even entered the room with the patient.* The behavioral specialist was then on hand to see the patient before, during, or immediately after the patient/provider encounter.

Based on this pattern, we asked our IT team to write a code that would automatically page the behavioral specialists as the patient completed the survey, even before the assistant greeted the patient in the waiting room, if the MCS score was 35 or less.

The key for us was not gathering more data. It was not harnessing variation to inspire change. Neither in isolation was enough. Understanding the process of care from a patient's perspective and visualizing how different microsystems had different processes was the key. Until we got to that point, nothing worked.

MICROSYSTEMS

A microsystem is where change occurs, no matter where the inspiration for the change originated, so it is important that we pay careful attention to defining the microsystem, the data it will need, and understand its patterns and opportunities, as well as its decision-making processes. Simply put, a microsystem is the smallest replicable unit needed to complete a task. The unit always consists of people doing the work, data about the work, and the end user. The end user in healthcare is a patient. All too often, project teams fail to consider "data" and "patient" as part of their project team.

A fast food restaurant is an example of a microsystem. There is a customer who is hungry and is greeted by a worker who takes the customer's order and completes the purchasing process. After taking the order, the worker conveys the data to another worker who makes the food item and a third worker who gathers the disparate food and drink items. In this simple example, the microsystem consists of the customer, data, and three workers. Understanding the smallest replicable unit and what it requires in order to function well makes it possible to string several together side by side and create a restaurant. It is then possible to replicate the design many times over to create thousands of restaurants.

An example of a healthcare system could consist of a patient with a persistent backache, a receptionist, a medical assistant, a physician, a physical therapist, and a behavioral health specialist.

ESSENTIAL PROCESS MAPPING

Process mapping in healthcare involves taking a patient perspective and recording each step needed to complete a process. This can be done by patients, as described earlier in this chapter. A third-party observer can also do it. It is an acquired skill to be able to observe but not interfere, and to bring a fresh eye to the situation, free of preconceptions. It is generally unwise to have leaders or staff from within the microsystem complete the observations because their familiarity and biases can lead them to miss important aspects of routine processes. This is why a small cluster of two to three trained observers can be so valuable to an entire organization's transformation efforts. At each step along the process, the observer notes the location, the task being completed, the title of those involved (MD, PT, NP, etc.) and the time required.

The following is a generic example of a single encounter between a patient
and a physician.

FIGURE: 5.1 PATIENT/PHYSICIAN ENCOUNTER PROCESS MAP

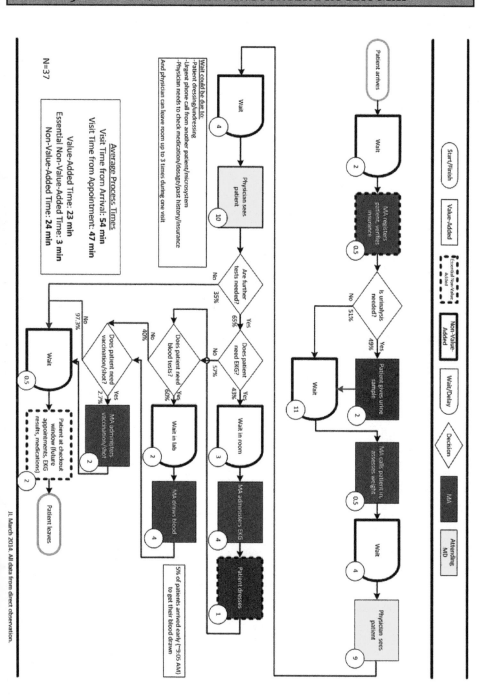

JL March 2014, All data from direct observation.

Different colors and shapes can be used to convey context, but they are not essential. In fact, it helps to keep things as simple as possible. The following, too, is an example of a typical office visit where the patient arrives, the nurse calls the patient into the exam room and asks the patient to complete a survey regarding his general health perception, and then the doctor sees the patient and the patient leaves with his need met.

FIGURE 5.2: THE CURRENT PROCESS

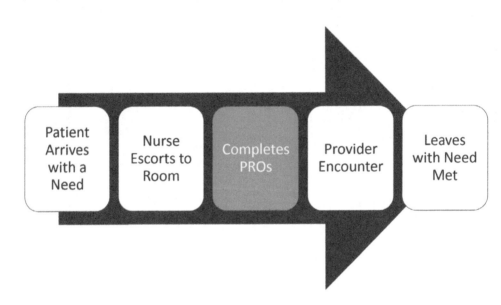

After the current process is mapped, we ask four questions:

1. How can this process be done better for the patient?

2. Is there a better or less expensive location for this process?

3. Are we using all the training and skills within our team to best address the patient's needs?

4. How can this process be done in less time for the patient?

Make the process better for the patient by looking for less expensive or more convenient locations where certain steps can occur, less expensive personnel who are able to complete tasks, and less expensive supplies and other resources that may be available. Look to remove steps that are redundant or unnecessary. Like items in a drawer, clutter happens to processes left unattended. Removing duplicate and unused items leads to less time wasted trying to find necessary items. Removing waste improves effectiveness and efficiency. Changing the order in which steps occur for the patient can also increase efficiency.

From our earlier, simplified example, we notice it would be possible to rearrange the process so the patient is completing the general health survey before entering the clinic. This keeps more exam rooms "in play" and helps to increase efficiency throughout the clinic.

FIGURE 5.3: THE NEW PROCESS

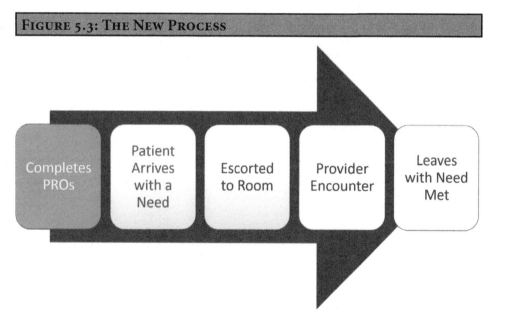

At this point it is wise to test the new process with small pilot where select staff "test drive" for a short amount of time (e.g., one week) the proposed process, including routines needed for any new measurements. After the pilot is complete, the participating staff debriefs, resulting data are analyzed, lessons learned are gathered and disseminated, and the process is revised as necessary. One or two pilot periods can be very helpful, but more than that are not.

COMPARE OLD TO NEW

Now that we have an old and a new process, we can compare outcomes that matter: quality, time, satisfaction (patient and staff), and costs. We reflect on our four basic process questions. How can we do this better? Is there a better or less expensive location? Are we using everyone's skill set to the top of his or her qualifications? How can we do this in less time? Assessing the impact of your effort requires comparing the outcomes and costs seen in the old process to those produced by the new process. In the next chapter we will go over some helpful tips on making those comparisons.

RESOURCES

» Quinn, J.B. (1992) *Intelligent Enterprise*. New York, NY: Free Press.

» Nelson, E.C., Batalden, P.B., & Godfrey, M.M. (2007). *Quality by Design*. San Francisco, CA: Jossey-Bass.

» Nelson, E.C., Batalden, P., Godfrey, M.M., & Lazar, J.S. (2011). *Value by Design*. San Francisco, CA: Jossey-Bass.

» Walsh. T. & Nelson, W.A. (2014) Ensuring patient-centered care. *The Healthcare Executive*. 29, 4.

» Nelson, W.A., Taylor, E., & Walsh, T. (2014) Leadership and transition: Building an ethical organizational culture. *The Health Care Manager*. 33, 3.

» Brownlee, S., Colucci, J., & Walsh, T. (2012) What "health care costs" really means. *The Atlantic Magazine*. (http://www.theatlantic.com/health/archive/2012/12/what-health-care-costs-really-means/266522/).

CHAPTER 6

DEMONSTRATING GREATER VALUE

Is the Signal Greater Than the Noise?

Healthcare teams are interested in learning which of their innovations has led to meaningful improvement, but conducting rigorous experiments in clinical settings is difficult because healthcare providers organize their clinics to care for patients as they arrive, regardless of where they have come from, their personal or cultural backgrounds, or their ability to pay.

These factors, and others, affect the health status of individuals arriving for care and their ability to respond to treatment, making it difficult to rigorously assess the impact of an intervention.

Unique Context

In addition, each clinic is unique in its own right, with differing proportions of patients from diverse backgrounds and social contexts. It is not only the patients that differ from one clinic to another; providers, administrators, and staff bring their own backgrounds, skill level, degree of interest in their patients, willingness to play an active role in improvement projects, along with their various levels of resilience and adaptability. More still, there are differences in how well clinical teams relate with one another and coordinate with other teams. Many of the things that make patients and clinics unique are difficult to measure or infrequently collected in databases, and as such, they go unmeasured.

Unknown Unknowns

Unmeasured variables are the gremlins that impair our ability to be confident about the generalizability of research findings as well as the results we see after implementing a new care process. Unmeasured variables can influence patients' health and their ability to respond to treatment as well as quality of care provided, so we must be cautious about claims that a new intervention is the sole cause of the outcomes we see day to day.

Unmeasured variables continually exert their hidden influence. The normal variations from moment to moment in each of the known and unknown variables combine to influence the health outcomes and quality of care for any patient. Because of these, there is always a range of outcomes around the average overall performance of a healthcare team. The range of outcomes surrounding the average creates the "noise" of a system, like the static out of a radio.

The Noise and a Signal

Each system's noise is unique. A healthcare team launches a new treatment, or begins using a redesigned care pathway, with the hope that it will improve health outcomes and/or improve team performance. Positive and substantial changes that are meaningful to patients, or the team, "signal" true improvement.

Ultimately, assessing whether or not an intervention improved the delivery of healthcare comes down to answering the question: Is the signal greater than the noise?

Statistical Analysis

At this point, readers thinking ahead may be anticipating a discussion of statistical techniques to analyze outcomes while looking for a significant difference. They would be wrong. **Analyses** of that type can only account for variables that are measured. However, the key to truly knowing the effect of an intervention lies in the **methods** used to address the unmeasured variables that make up a system's noise.

Of course, statistical analyses are valuable and can provide insight, but analytic techniques are not the focus here. As you will see, it is possible to assess the effect of an intervention in healthcare delivery using only subtraction and clinical awareness.

Analysis cannot make up for an inadequate method. Unmeasured variables will bias the assessment of an intervention if the correct methods are not used. There are three methods for eliminating the bias of unmeasured variables. The best method is to create two groupings—an intervention group and a control group, and randomly assign people and/or places to the intervention group or the control group. Randomization is best because it will equally allocate the unmeasured variables to both groups, mitigating any biases that would influence the intervention's effects.

Occasionally, a variable will share these features of the randomization process. That is, it will determine group assignment and equally allocate unmeasured variables to both groups, but it will have no additional influence on the effects created by the intervention. Variables that can function like randomization are called instrumental variables. An everyday example of a randomizing process is a coin-flip. In healthcare, things that can sometimes act like a coin-flip include program eligibility that varies by geography (think, Medicaid) or the distance to a treatment facility. They are not common, but when found, they are magical for research scientists. Instrumental variables, then, can be likened to gnomes—they have magical powers, but good ones are difficult to find.

Measuring the impact of our interventions, then, can be a challenge. Many statistical techniques—from multivariate and multi-level regression, to propensity scores, to regression discontinuity—are attempts to find the signal among the noise. These techniques cannot make up for the unmeasured variables we have been discussing. This is not to say they are not useful, but it is important to recognize their limitations. Additional techniques for monitoring change in processes over time—called Statistical Process Control assessments—can also be helpful. Moreover, SPCs are useful to monitor a system's performance in real time. SPCs will be explored in more detail later in the chapter.

A MORE PRACTICAL WAY

Randomization is not always practical and instrumental variables are hard to find. Fortunately, there is a third, more practical, way to find the true signal from our intervention over the usual system noise. The practical method requires a baseline assessment of the system's functioning and process outcomes. Trained third-party observers are best for this because they can more easily blend in and have less influence on normal functioning, whereas a large influence is produced if a senior leader does the observation. Through baseline observation, it is possible to utilize a "difference in differences" method to identify an unbiased signal. In other words, with baseline data a practical way exists to assess the real impact of your intervention. This practical method for dealing with unobserved variables works on those variables that remain stable over time. Let's walk through an example to demonstrate the calculations.

A DIFFERENCE IN DIFFERENCES

Many healthcare teams would like to assess the impact of an intervention to improve their delivery of healthcare using a mental model like the one shown below, where the launch of the intervention also marks the beginning of data collection. The effect of the intervention is estimated by finding the difference between the group receiving the intervention ("I") compared to the group that did not receive the intervention, or the Control Group ("C").

FIGURE 6.1: COMMON EVALUATION TECHNIQUE

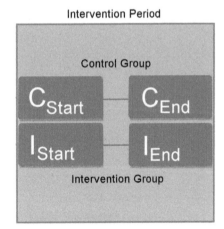

A Common Evaluation Technique

Intervention Period

Control Group

C_{Start} — C_{End}

I_{Start} — I_{End}

Intervention Group

Effect = (X)

$(I_{End} - I_{Start}) - (C_{End} - C_{Start})$

Arbitrary numbers can illustrate how the calculation unfolds. At the end of the intervention period, the control group improved by 3 points and the intervention group improved by 10. The effect of our intervention then appears to be 7 points.

The key point, however, is to remember we have no way of knowing if the unmeasured variables are equally spread between both the intervention and control groups. This means our estimation of the effect may be biased.

FIGURE 6.2: BIASED EVALUATION TECHNIQUE

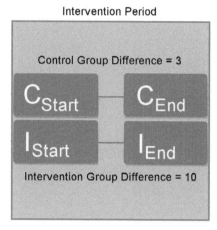

A ~~Common~~ Evaluation Technique

A Biased

x = 7

Intervention Period

Control Group Difference = 3

C_{Start} — C_{End}

I_{Start} — I_{End}

Intervention Group Difference = 10

Effect = (X)
(10) - (3)

The use of a baseline period is the most practical way for healthcare teams to remove bias from their assessment of an intervention. Finding the average change in outcomes experienced by all participants during the baseline period, then subtracting that from the effect found in the comparison of the intervention and control groups removes the bias so long as no other changes occurred between the baseline and intervention periods. The next figure uses arbitrary numbers to show the calculations.

FIGURE 6.3: UNBIASED EVALUATION TECHNIQUE

An Unbiased Evaluation Technique

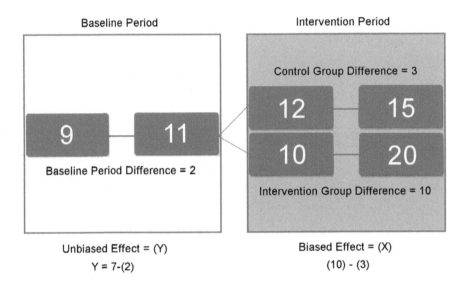

In this example, we see that noise in the system creates its own change of two points under everyday conditions. Removing the noise provides us with better insight into the change produced by our intervention. Recall, in our initial, noisy, estimate of change shown above was seven points - At the end of the intervention period, the control group improved by 3 points and the intervention group improved by 10. The effect of our intervention then appeared to be 7 points. However, with careful observation during the baseline period we learned that our current system produced a change of two points.

The two point change seen in our current system should not be attributed to our intervention, so we subtract those two points from the effect of the intervention, lowering the improvement from 10 to 8 points. This means the true signal created by the intervention was five points. Now we can ask: "Is five a big change?"

FIGURE 6.4: UNBIASED EVALUATION METHODOLOGY

An Unbiased Evaluation Technique

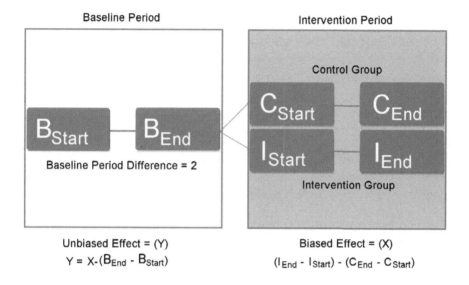

Baseline Period

Intervention Period

Control Group

C_{Start} C_{End}

B_{Start} B_{End}

I_{Start} I_{End}

Baseline Period Difference = 2

Intervention Group

Unbiased Effect = (Y)

$Y = X - (B_{End} - B_{Start})$

Biased Effect = (X)

$(I_{End} - I_{Start}) - (C_{End} - C_{Start})$

SIGNIFICANT VS. MEANINGFUL

Statisticians can perform tests to determine statistical significance, but not all statistically significant changes are clinically meaningful. Here is another way to ask these questions:

» Would you alter your work based on a change of that magnitude?

» Would a patient find the change meaningful?

The most important thing you can do to strengthen your assessment of the impact made by a change is to have pre-intervention data as a baseline group. The difference in differences method is impossible without baseline data acting as a control group. This can be accomplished using an interrupted time series or a phased-in approach across multiple sites where late adapters serve as controls for early implementers, something that is very much in the realm of possibility for multi-hospital systems.

This may all seem like a lot of bother, but given the substantial costs associated with many transformation efforts and the data infrastructure they require, leaders deciding to adopt an improvement project should demand more exacting evaluations.

In moving from the discussion of methods to analytic techniques, it's important to consider what is wanted from them. We would like techniques that are as simple as can be, with minimal chance for misinterpretation, close to real-time as possible, and explainable in common terms. Statistical process control is an analytic approach meeting these criteria and it has proven useful for assessing organizational change. The SPC approach displays variation so researchers, administrators, healthcare providers, and patients can better understand the impact of transformation efforts. Healthcare SPC authority, Dr. Raymond G. Carey, has defined SPC as "...*a philosophy, a strategy, and a set of techniques for ongoing improvement of systems, processes, and outcomes. The SPC approach is based on learning through data and has its foundation in the theory of variation (understanding common and special causes).*"

The key to understanding SPC comes from realizing all processes have their own variation. Some processes exhibit a small amount of variation, while some will exhibit a considerable amount. Some processes exhibit stable variation, be it small or great, while the variation in others is unstable. Observe a process long enough and you can find its variation signature. Maybe the process speeds up on Tuesdays and slows down when Dr. Smith is involved. Tuesdays and Dr. Smith are common causes of variation—they contribute to the natural variation for this process. A special cause of variation refers to perturbations inflicted on the process by uncommon circumstances.

Continuing with our example, imagine a special case where for one week Dr. Smith switches from his typical schedule and works on a Tuesday. We would expect to see an uncommonly slow process that Tuesday because of this special case. Seeing the uncommon slowdown in productivity on that particular Tuesday, we would investigate why Dr. Smith switched days, and we might learn that the clinician who usually works on Tuesday is on vacation.

In this manner, we can observe the variation of any process, learn its common causes, predict the amount of expected variation created by the common causes, and investigate special causes further. We may find some processes that exhibit special causes of variation all the time. Their pattern of variation is unstable and the process is unpredictable. The first step, then, is to observe the process in its natural state, while looking for ways to standardize the work enough to gain some stability and predictability.

Once a process is stable, it is possible to predict a range of expected variation for the future. Furthermore, it is possible to establish both upper and lower limits for the expected variation and to then analyze any change in variation for statistical evidence of change. These properties allow us to create charts plotting process performance against time. The body of the chart will be divided by three lines: one indicating a chosen measure at each point in time, another indicating the upper limit, and the third indicating the lower limit. Consider this example charting the number of emergency room visits for patients with diabetes. Patients with well controlled diabetes should not need emergency care, but the chart shows month to month variation in the number of admissions ranging from a high of 14 in August of year 1 to a single admission in October of year 3.

FIGURE 6.5: CONTROL CHART WITH UPPER AND LOWER LIMITS

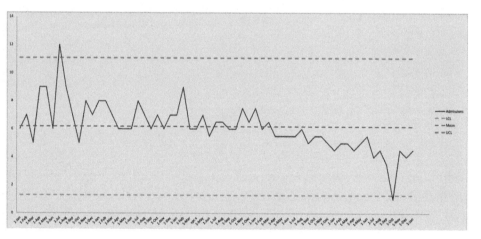

By convention, the upper and lower limits are set at +/- 3 standard deviations around the mean produced by the process because this is felt to be a pragmatic compromise between setting limits too tightly, which leads to erroneous conclusions regarding the predictability of the data, or too loosely, where the risk is missing important information. The formula used to calculate the standard deviation is different for different types of data. The most common types of data used in healthcare processes are those with which it is possible to calculate an average, categories where it is possible to calculate proportions, and events where we want to measure the period between them. Examples of these three types include the average wait time a patient spends in an exam room without seeing a provider, the proportion of patients with a positive depression screening who are assessed by a behavioral medicine specialist, and the number of days between significant, but infrequent events like a patient falling down Regardless of the method for calculating the data limits, points above or below the limit lines represent special cause variation.

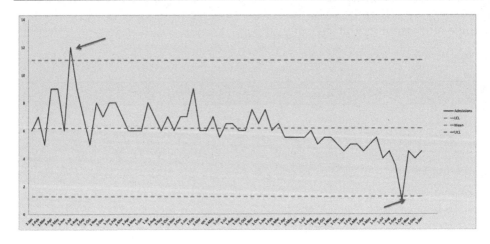

FIGURE 6.6: SPECIAL CAUSE VARIATION IDENTIFIED BY DATA POINTS OUTSIDE OF LIMIT LINES

Additional rules for identifying special cause variation have been developed and include spotting trends, like eight or more data points on the same side of the centerline as seen on the far right of the figure above.

SPC charts are easy for clinicians, administrators, patients, and C-suite leaders to understand, but they are not simple to correctly construct. This is why data engineers are so important for an organization. One person, well trained, can advise several project leaders regarding the appropriate methods and the best analytic techniques for assessing the impact of transformation efforts.

By the way, these charts depicting emergency admissions for patients with diabetes created a lot of dialogue and initial worry. Through careful investigation, we came to understand the spike in august of year 1 was due to primary care providers taking vacation time and patients eating less carefully. We were able adjust staffing accordingly and our show improvement. The lowest number of admissions occurred in year 3, during October when most providers were back from vacation.

RESOURCES

» White, H. (2006). Impact Evaluation. *The experience of the independent evaluation group of the World Bank.* Washington, DC: World Bank.

» Ravallion, M. (2001). The mystery of the vanishing benefits: An introduction to impact evaluation. *The World Bank Economic Review* 2001. 15(1),115-140.

» Vest, J.R., & Gamm, L.D. (2009). A critical review of the research literature on six sigma, lean, and Studer Group's hardwiring excellence in the United States: The need to demonstrate and communicate the effectiveness of transformation strategies in healthcare. *Implementation Science.* 4, 35.

» Carey, R. (2003) *Improving healthcare with control charts: basic and advanced SPC methods and case studies.* Milwaukee: ASQ Quality Press.

» Institute for Healthcare Improvement. Run Chart Tool. http:// www. ihi.org/knowledge/Pages/Tools/RunChart.aspx

» Thor, J., Lundberg, J., Ask, J., Olsson J,. Carli, C., Harenstam, K.P., & Brommels, M. Application of statistical process control in healthcare: A systematic review. *Qual Saf Health Care.*16, 387-399

CHAPTER 7

COMMUNICATING AND COORDINATING TO CREATE GREATER VALUE THROUGHOUT AN ORGANIZATION

COMMUNICATING AND COORDINATING

During my eight years at the Dartmouth-Hitchcock Spine Center, I had the opportunity to lead improvement projects and conduct clinical research. One of the improvement projects was meant to improve access for patients coming to the spine center. It failed miserably because of poor communication and coordination.

Many of the senior providers at the spine center considered a long waiting list of patients to be a sign of respect from referring providers and a signal of unmet need for their services. Meanwhile, a small core of us wanted to improve access to better meet our patients' needs and to increase enrollment in our research. We met regularly and searched the literature on operations management, queuing theory applied to healthcare settings, and workflow analysis. We learned the value of monitoring the third next available appointment (see *http://www.ihi.org/resources/Pages/Measures/ThirdNextAvailableAppointment.aspx*) and calculated ours, which was nearly 22 days. The recommended third next available appointment timeframe for primary care is zero and two days for specialty care. Our cloistered group had its work cut out. All of us agreed. We drafted an outstanding plan.

We unveiled our plan to the wider group at a monthly all-staff meeting. I could be accused of exaggerating if I told you it was met with hisses, boos, and thrown vegetables—and I would be exaggerating, but just barely.

It turns out the clear majority of people do not like to have their schedules altered without being consulted.

It should have been obvious ahead of time. It is something that everybody knows intuitively—attempting to impose a change upon one or more people will lead to resistance. If you have enough authority, you can do it and see short-term success, but at the cost of deteriorating commitment, trust and engagement.

If everyone knows this, why does it keep happening? Many transformation efforts have failed because of "poor communication." For example, another innovation center determined physician efficiency could be improved by installing new office furniture—exam tables that could transition from chair to table and back. One weekend, several chairs were installed in exam rooms and the old furniture was donated away. It took only three patient encounters to realize there were no arm rests on the chairs, which meant it was nearly impossible for some patients to sit down or get up safely. A nurse, a doctor, or an assistant needed to safely transfer patients. Also concerning was the lack of a spool to hold exam table paper that needed to be changed between each patient. Not only was there nothing to hold it, once the patient was seated it was impossible to place the paper over the length of the exam table. The exam paper had to be stored in a cupboard and then retrieved, as the patient was about to recline for the exam. But first, the patient needed to stand up again, which meant he or she needed assistance, which was hardly an improvement in efficiency.

Making sure your communication plan includes end users—clinicians, receptionists, and patients—is critical.

Before you begin an improvement project consider who needs to know and how to keep them aware. Many projects lose momentum unnecessarily, and very good projects have been stymied because someone who should have known about the project or its processes did not. At a minimum, the project leader and the people implementing the change need to understand why the change is occurring and what is expected as a result. Furthermore, it is important to have a line of communication open between the project leader and those who will receive the benefits of the change—the end user, or most often in healthcare, the patient. Patient architects, described in the next section, can be helpful here.

Similarly, to prevent wasting time and energy, it is important to consider how you will communicate with organizational leaders in oversight roles. In times of limited funds, choices must made, and even an excellent idea may need to be shelved for a short period while other priorities are addressed. Better to know this early than to find out late.

PROJECT TEAM

The project team is where the change occurs; it's the proverbial "sharp end of the spear." The project team usually meets every one to two weeks to review outstanding action items and compare progress to the timeline. The team works together to address concerns when possible flag and true barriers for the steering and/or oversight committee to address. Successes are acknowledged and celebrated. The weekly project team meeting also has responsibilities for how action items are determined and dispensed.

STEERING COMMITTEE

Many organizations have steering committees. Steering committees typically include mid-level organizational leaders, data engineers, and patient architects who work to refine timeline expectations, anticipate leadership barriers, and maintain measurement focus. Barriers to progress are anticipated where possible, and identified barriers are addressed. Successes are recognized. The steering committee typically meets for each project phase and quarterly during a phase.

OVERSIGHT COMMITTEE

The oversight committee meets for each project phase and occasionally during mid implementation. Approval from an oversight committee is usually required before beginning any transformation project. In addition, the oversight committee meets to address newly identified barriers and to compare anticipated progress to reality for key measures, timeframes, and budgets.

Front-line team members doing the actual work create many of the best improvement initiatives. When that happens, it becomes necessary to communicate up to the organizational leadership. A little homework done regarding the members and priorities of the committee saves a lot of time. By the time someone has risen to the oversight level, he or she will have a public record of accomplishment. Reading their publicly available biographies will provide insight into their personal priorities. When possible, it is wise to find a member of the oversight committee with interests that match what you wish to accomplish. Oversight committees have organizational priorities as well. Understanding these and where the current project aligns with them is crucial because the committee will reject even great ideas if the timing and priorities do not match. The only way to overcome this roadblock is to develop a champion on the committee. This is always the result of doing your homework and building relationships with individuals who may one day spearhead your project.

Organization leaders, regardless of where the improvement initiative originates, will need to communicate right to up to the board, across organizational boundaries, as well as to everyone else involved in the enterprise. In most organizations, these types of activities occur in meetings.

Running a meeting, whether it is for a weekly project team or the oversight committee, takes communication skills. But outstanding communication skills alone are not sufficient in managing an improvement project, or leading an organization and more than they're sufficient for the care of chronically ill patients, However, in each case, poor communication skills will not only kill motivation, they will inspire resistance.

In many ways it is not unlike a series of clinic visits with a patient working to optimize his or her health in the face of a chronic condition. As with any other skill, communication skills improve with deliberate practice, whether with patients or with co-workers.

Words matter.

Presence matters.

Deliberately practicing to improve communication skills is vital.

Consider the healthcare provider who takes a moment to review her last visit with a patient who is struggling with several months of low back pain and co-morbid depression. She enters the encounter with the patient, and after the typical greeting, begins with, "The last time you were here, we discussed physical therapy for your back pain and cognitive behavioral therapy for your depression." The physician then pauses to check her patient's body language; is he nodding in agreement or looking confused as if he can't recall the prior conversation? She is gauging engagement.

Her next statement to the patient is a question, "Have you had a chance to try either or both of them?" If the answer is negative, her task will be helping the patient problem-solve so the desired actions are completed. If the answer is positive, her next questions seek to identify barriers she may be able to alleviate and successes that she can celebrate with her patient. She then moves on, in collaboration with the patient, to design a plan going forward. The best communicators will then ask the patient to "teach back" the plan. Meaning to describe their understanding of what should happen next. The very best communicators do not stop there. They go on to ask, "On a scale of zero to 10, with zero being no confidence at all and 10 being complete confidence, how confident are you that you can do the plan?" Any answer less than eight generates a follow-up: "What would it take to raise that score to an eight or nine?"

Now imagine the same patient returns one month later and our physician reviews her notes, greets the patient and begins with the following:

» The last time you were here we discussed…

» Have you had a chance to do it?

» What have you found?

» Can you show me how you will explain our plan going forward to your family?

» How confident are you about the plan

» What needs to happen for you to be very confident?

And the same questions are kindly asked at the next appointment.

While such a structured approach may seem awkward at first, the likelihood that such an approach will help the patient to implement the plan rises substantially. Expectations are being set clearly. There is respect and collaboration.

This same approach is similarly beneficial when running meetings to create greater value. The meeting leader prepares for the meeting and begins, "The last time we were here, we agreed on the following items." He then lists the items and who is responsible for each item while simultaneously checking body language. Then he asks for an update on each of the items. What barriers were encountered, what successes need to be celebrated, and what is needed going forward. Together, the meeting's attendees collaboratively plan next steps and seek to build confidence in the plan.

The key statements, actions, and questions for results-focused meetings are:

» "The last time we were here, we discussed…" and assess body language

» "Have you had a chance to try it?" and listen

» "What have you found?" and listen

» Collaboratively create a plan going forward

» Assess confidence in the plan directly by asking, "How confident are you about this plan?" and assess body language

» If needed, ask "What needs to happen for you to be very confident?" and assess body language

Meetings of the project team, steering committee, and oversight committee occur at regular intervals, which make it possible to create a rhythm to your communication. Organize your meeting rhythm to make the best use of everyone's time and energy because that attention, or lack of attention, to the details of your communication plan and cadence can make or break your project.

And like communication planning, there is also a cadence to the phases of implementing a change.

A Typical Project Timeline

Most projects will have four distinct phases—scoping, diagnostic, implementation, and sustainment.

Scoping

The scoping phase includes defining the problem the project will try to solve, and a high-level estimate on timeframes and budget. The diagnostic phase includes gathering information on the current status and the desired future status for a process. The gap between the current status and the future status will be used to create the tension that is necessary for change, will provide a vision for what success can realistically look like, and suggest first steps towards the envisioned end state.

DIAGNOSTIC

All systems are inherently resistant to change. Overcoming organizational inertia requires a degree of dissatisfaction with the status quo, a vision for something better, and winnable first steps to build momentum. The diagnostic phase is where you will build dissatisfaction, the vision, and define winnable first steps. It is also where you will begin thinking about measuring the current status and monitoring the change efforts. You'll start thinking about what metrics are best, where do those data live, who can retrieve, organize, and display the data in order to turn it into useful information. The diagnostic phase is also where more detailed timeline is developed for getting from the current state to the desired state.

IMPLEMENTATION

The implementation phase unfolds on the timeline first outlined in the diagnostic phase. Some aspects of the implementation plan will unfold differently than planned. Experience has shown that the normal life cycle for a project is longer than first imagined, harder than desired, and typically includes a crisis moment, or two. This is why agility and adaptability are key attributes of successful projects.

SUSTAINMENT

The sustainment phase is ongoing. Performance dashboards monitor are helpful here. Consider pilots, key measures needed for flight are displayed in a very easy to read way. Altitude, for instance, could be monitored by text placed on the ceiling near some switches. It is better, however, to have key measures thoughtfully selected and placed on a performance dashboard where quick glances can let us answer the question: Are they improving, sustaining, or degrading? What needs to happen to ensure continued success? What lessons have been learned and how will they be communicated to help others fail faster and succeed more efficiently?

The table on the following page shows the rhythm for a typical communication plan across implementation phases.

FIGURE 7.1: MEETING RHYTHM CHART

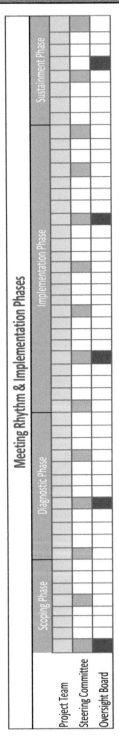

CHAPTER 8

ATTRIBUTES OF SUCCESSFUL TRANSFORMATIONS TO VALUE

Successful Transformations to Value

Back in Northern New York State the paper forms we were using to survey patients about their pain and function were piling up, and our practice was growing. The anxiety-filled lunches and gloomy outlook were replaced by a sense of accomplishment and the realization that times were changing - for the better! As we grew from one clinic to four, we made a point of teaching each clinic how to distribute and collect the forms. We taught all new clinical staff to review the forms with each patient and to look for patterns among their patients. We did not know it at the time, but our team, through luck alone, possessed many attributes that would later prove essential for transforming the practice. We were truly a team. Any one of us could lead when necessary and follow when it seemed best. We all felt that our individual efforts made a difference. We had the support of the organization (we led it) and we had a learning, rather than a blaming, mindset.

Later in my career, as a result of several frustrating experiences trying to implement changes, I wanted to learn what I could do to better ensure a project's success. It turns out there are several key attributes to successful transformation efforts. I lucked out with my first effort, but I have since learned how to be more mindful about creating fertile ground before expecting a bountiful harvest.

While in many ways a single person can make a profound difference in the world, it is hard to transform healthcare delivery alone. It takes a team and organizational commitment, but a team of senior leaders cannot mandate successful transformation. It requires engaged people at all levels of the organization. Moreover, it requires an organizational appreciation of the road ahead. The road leads to better value for patients, providers, payers, businesses, and communities, but the work required to get there is often underappreciated.

To get a sense of how underappreciated transformation and improvement projects are, just ask someone about innovation in healthcare. Invariably, he or she will tell you about new technology—a new device, new drug, maybe a new surgical technique. The lack of appreciation for the innovation brought by improvement efforts has meant that they have been poorly understood and misused. This becomes clear when a director of graduate medical education says she is "always happy" when a resident picks "raise our lung cancer or colorectal cancer screening rate," as his or her improvement project "because we can always make those numbers go back up." Statements like that reveal a gross conceptual error in thinking about improvement. If your organization sees a need to continually revisit the same past projects, and finds a need to repeat the effort, you are ultimately failing—despite being able to demonstrate improvement once again.

Due to their haphazard use, improvement efforts have been under-researched. Rather than having systematic reviews of what works best and how to do it, we have hard-won knowledge of how difficult it is to generalize findings from one organization to another. Emerging from those ashes, there is some consensus regarding what is needed in order to avoid past mistakes. What then, are the attributes of successful transformation efforts?

Successful transformation is typically a series of sequential improvement efforts focused on improving the value of care in high-cost areas, such as the treatment of patients with long-term low back pain, then applying the lessons learned across the organization. As successes mount, the organization is transformed into an agile, adaptable, receptive delivery system capable of demonstrably creating value. . The work is done by teams, so it is appropriate to begin by examining the attributes of successful project teams, their leaders, and the ways that organizations can support their efforts.

THE PROJECT TEAM

The ability to work collaboratively has traditionally been underappreciated and, many times, undervalued by organizations. This is changing and it is a good thing because rigid, hierarchical, authoritarian types suppress input from end users, just as authoritarian physicians squelch patients from contributing to their own treatment plans. In both circumstances, insights needed for increasing value are lost.

The best team members are those who:

> » Are agile–the type that can switch from an assertive, highly organized "Type A" to more relaxed, somewhat lassiez-faire "Type B" and back as needed.

» Have an ability to adapt quickly in a dynamic environment

» Have a sense of personal empowerment—a belief that his or her effort can make a difference.

PROJECT LEADERSHIP

Project leaders who are most likely to succeed have an ability to develop working relationships with senior leaders across the boundaries created by departments and hierarchies. They seek out and value input from all team members, not just that of their peers or anyone senior. They are also adept at developing working relationships with data managers and have working knowledge of analytic techniques.

ORGANIZATIONAL LEADERSHIP

The most frequently cited feature of organizational leadership associated with successful transformation is accessibility. Transformative leaders visibly define successful outcomes and align their organization's actions and ethics. In addition, they make every effort to provide high-quality personnel to improvement efforts. In short, the leaders of organizations that have made successful transformations enable, encourage, and support improvement efforts in ways that are visible to every employee.

ORGANIZATIONAL SUPPORT

One efficient and effective way to enable, encourage, and support improvement efforts is by creating centralized units committed to the transformation process across departmental boundaries. This facilitates the growth of institutional knowledge so that "lessons learned" from work done in orthopedics, for example, are understood and are drawn upon for a project about to begin in palliative care. A typical staff within a centralized unit includes a cluster of experienced coaches. The coaches are people within the organization who have participated in prior efforts and have the energy and interest to mentor others. The coaches typically have full-time positions in their home departments, so it is up to the organization to support their coaching efforts by allowing them to take time for their mentoring activity. This is no small request given the salaries of surgeons, physicians, and senior administrators, but organizations that have successfully transformed find a way to do it. The payoff is difficult to quantify, but faster learning cycles can lead to effective changes occurring more quickly. Most organizations believe the eight or so hours per month devoted to mentoring is a bargain. The center's staff also contains data engineers with expertise in retrieving, organizing, and displaying data in order to create actionable information for project teams, steering committees and senior leader oversight. A single data engineer can work with multiple projects simultaneously because projects are not synchronized (i.e., the bulk of work occurs during the early phases of a project and it is rare to have multiple transformation projects starting at the same time).

Experienced third-party observers have also proven very helpful. Trained in anthropology or sociology, their skills are important for process mapping, ethnographic interviews, and documenting communication skills. The ability to observe without being obtrusive takes practice and few leaders have the time or desire to master it. Like data engineers, a single trained third-party observer can work with multiple projects simultaneously.

Transformation centers benefit from having patients on staff to advocate for the patient's perspective. Most hospitals, clinics, and processes are structured for efficient throughput and the staff's comfort, and in structuring this way have failed to appreciate and address the patient experience. For this reason, it is important for the center to maintain a small cadre of patients whom it consults regularly. An appropriate title for the patient's position can help demonstrate the importance of their role. Some have found Patient Architect, a term coined by the Connecticut Institute for Primary Care Innovation, serves this purpose nicely.

The basic unit for an organization's Transformation Center, then, is a mentor, a data engineer, a third-party observer and a patient architect. Over time, the center becomes the holder of organizational knowledge regarding transformation efforts—what has worked, what has not, and why. This increases the pace of all subsequent efforts.

MINDSET AND EXPECTATIONS

While there is much to learn from improvement efforts elsewhere, each project will have its own unique context and no comprehensive answer exists for all the challenges to be faced during a given transformation effort. This makes generalizing from another organization's efforts difficult, even those of an esteemed organization, and especially of an esteemed organization's prior work. There is much to learn from past pioneers, but transformation efforts occur in complex and adapting systems that are different from simple or even complicated systems and are unique to every setting.

Simple systems encounter problems that have simple, reproducible answers. A good example might be making a sandwich. The process is straightforward, as are its attendant problems, like a lack of resources (you're out of bread), which can be fixed quickly. After making many sandwiches, it is easy to reach a point where a consistent product is produced.

Complicated systems—landing a rover on Mars, for example—involve many more steps, and the problems that come up can be significant. However, once it has been done, you can have a high degree of confidence that doing the same steps in the same order will produce the same results.

Complex systems are more dynamic and involved than either simple or complicated systems. Raising children is a good example here. There are so many variables and they are adapting to one another and changing one another so much that it becomes difficult to tease out cause and effect. The results are not predictable. A good outcome with one, two, or even three in no way ensures the next will be similar. In complex systems, similar to families raising multiple children, the best mindset is one of iterative, experiential discovery. There are things that can be done to decrease the likelihood of being led to faulty conclusions due to unseen biases, confounding variables, and chance, but in complex systems you discover from experience over and over again.

SUMMARY OF THE ATTRIBUTES OF SUCCESSFUL IMPROVEMENT EFFORTS

» Project team—The best team members are agile, able to adapt quickly in a dynamic environment and have a sense of person empowerment—a belief that his or her effort will make a difference

» Project leadership—The best project leaders are able to develop working relationships across boundaries. They value, and seek out, input from all team members as well as senior leaders. In addition, project leaders must be able to develop working relationships with and working knowledge of data management and analysis techniques.

» Organizational leadership—The best organizational leaders are accessible and work to align an organization's actions and ethics.

They provide high-quality personnel and time to the improvement efforts and work to enable, encourage and support improvement efforts.

» Organizational support—Organizations that figure out how to manage rapid change will thrive. Creating a small, centralized cluster of experienced coaches, data engineers and patient architects maximizes adaptability by building shared knowledge of what works locally.

» Mindset and Expectation—The best mindset for this work comes from an appreciation of complex system dynamics and learning by doing.

RESOURCES

»   Useem, M. (2001) *Leading Up*. New York, NY: Three Rivers Press.

»   Batalden, P. *Leading the improvement of healthcare*. http://www.sheffieldmca.org.uk/UserFiles/File/Batalden_1_page_book_1.pdf

»   Fussell, C.L., Hough, T. & Pedersen, M.D. (2009) *What Makes Fusion Cells Effective?* Monterey, CA: Naval Postgraduate School.

CHAPTER 9

EXAMPLES OF TRANSFORMATIONS THAT WORK IN CREATING VALUE

In the figure below, the horizontal, x-axis represents illness severity, with more severity found the further you go to the right. The vertical, or y-axis, shows both harms and benefits of a treatment. It could be any treatment. The light gray line represents harms. As you can see, the potential harm from any treatment is roughly similar regardless of illness severity. The side effects, for example, of a medication can occur to anyone who takes it, whether he or she is well or sick, so the line is fairly flat. Benefits, however, become greater. A very sick person restored to health will report a large benefit from a treatment while a less sick person receiving the same treatment would report less benefit. That person had less room to improve. The benefit line slopes up.

The interesting thing happens where the lines cross. Theoretically, a well person given a treatment can only experience the harmful side effects. If we think about it, this makes sense. Giving healthy people a treatment with side effects cannot make them healthier. It can only lead to harm. Meanwhile, on the far right, very sick patients are receiving tremendous benefit that far outweighs any harmful side effects.

Realize that only a very few people are in the set are "the most sick." The top figure simply shows how few people are in the far end of a distribution—where the sickest patients, who experience the greatest benefit from treatment, are to be found.

FIGURE 9.1: THE HOT SPOT

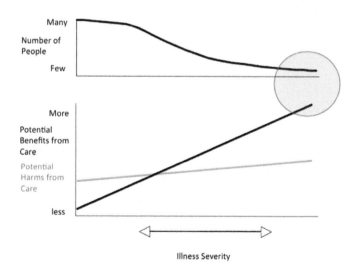

Illness Severity

How it Works

The sickest patients are where the benefits of treatment far outweigh the potential harms. Finding your sickest patients, identifying the intervention(s) they need (it may or may not be healthcare), and then successfully getting it to them is what hotspotting is about. It works because the net benefit is so large. At points of less illness severity, some of the net benefit is negated by the harmful side effects.

In this book, I have mentioned several medical processes where focused improvement efforts have led to measureable improvements in patient outcomes and/or cost lowering efforts, (i.e., they have proven to be quick successes). These include spine surgeries, hip and knee replacements, the elective induction of preterm births, stenting for blocked arteries of the heart, concurrent hospice care for patients with a terminal diagnosis. Hotspotting is relevant to each of them. Who are the patients with a compromised spine, joints, heart, or immune system and whose function is declining? Finding them, listening to them describe their needs, and interpreting what matters most to them will inform care providers about what needs to be done to prevent further decline. Many times, what is needed is not more healthcare, but better support for daily tasks and for family members. For this reason, paying attention to how your healthcare services integrate with community resources can pay big dividends.

Some organizations spend considerable amounts of money to purchase tools to help clinicians identify patients at the highest risk of becoming hospitalized or otherwise incurring great costs. Leaders of those organizations should not forget their most valuable hotspotting resource, their own nurses.

Resources

» *Jeff Brenner's Approach to Improving Health Care Delivery.* https://www.youtube.com/watch?v=id06Y-P58UE

» *How "Hot Spotting" Cut Health Care Costs.* The Robert Wood Johnson Foundation. http://www.rwjf.org/en/about-rwjf/ newsroom/features-and-articles/Brenner11.html

» *Building a hotspotting analytic toolkit.* http://www.camdenhealth. org/building-a-hotspotting-toolkit/

Integrating Behavioral Health in Care Pathway
What it is

Evidence from hotspotting, and extending back many years before that term was invented, along with clinical observation and common sense all tell us that patients with the greatest disease burden—those on the far right hotspotting scale—have multiple comorbidities. Co-morbid adjustment disorders like anxiety and depression, as well as mental illnesses like schizophrenia, can make it difficult for an individual to behave in ways that promote good health.

Evidence also suggests that co-morbid adjustment disorders remain under-diagnosed and under-treated. A behavioral health specialist established in a primary-care setting promotes increased recognition of the problem, raises treatment rates, and decreases hospitalizations and readmissions. Experiments with embedding primary-care providers in behavioral health settings is also showing promise. Screening for adjustment disorders in specialty care using patient reported measures can also help increase the recognition and treatment of co-morbid depression.

How it Works

Integration of behavioral health specialists and primary care—regardless of who visits whose home clinic—works because behavioral approaches, like cognitive behavioral therapy for treating anxiety and depression, are effective. As the burden of anxiety, depression, or similar conditions begins to lighten, patients are better able to care for their physical well-being. This is true whether the condition consist of spinal aliments, joint arthropathies, cardiovascular disease, or terminal diagnoses.

In the first few years of the Spine Center at Dartmouth Hitchcock Medical Center, patients became accustomed to answering general health questionnaires using a laptop. As we became more familiar with recognizing patterns in the dashboard display, it appeared that a higher than expected percentage of the patients had self-reported mental status and emotional well-being falling below the age- and gender-adjusted normal values. At first, being academics, we argued about which came first, the spinal problem or the emotional problem. After months of that, we questioned whether the general survey was actually signaling something or was merely reflecting something normal for patients with chronic pain. After all, many of the symptoms of chronic pain, including lethargy and a decreased desire to pursue activities, are also common symptoms of depression.

To investigate, we embedded a depression-specific survey that was developed precisely for use with patients who also had chronic pain. For several months, every patient completed both the general health survey we had always used and the depression-specific survey chosen for this investigation. We found that, indeed, our patients were reporting depressive symptoms beyond anything expected from chronic pain alone. Over time, we were able to use statistical techniques to identify what score on the general health survey best predicted a positive depression screen. We could then remove the depression-specific survey to keep the response burden as low as possible.

This process was not ideal. Other clinicians, not the behavioral specialist, were not comfortable discussing a patient's mood. They had no training in how to begin the conversation and no understanding regarding what to do if the conversation "went south" or somehow got beyond their comfort zone.

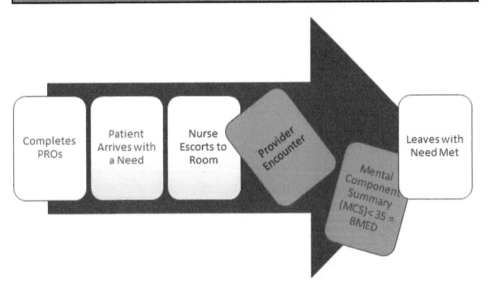

FIGURE 9.2: REFERRAL PROCESS FOR BEHAVIORAL MEDICINE FELL APART WHEN LEFT TO OTHER CLINICIANS

It was difficult for the behavioral specialist because the system interrupted his work and he then had to juggle what he had been doing with seeing an unscheduled patient. The process was successful, however, in addressing what had been an unrecognized, substantial problem. There were other problems with this system as well. For example, billing was complicated. Both the behavioral specialist's impromptu visit and the planned encounter with a specialist occurred occasionally at the same time. How do you bill for that? It turns out that you can but the procedure is different for every payer and the procedure changes every year or so.

None of that has anything to do with whether behavioral therapy was the right thing for the patient at that time. As it turns out, it was. Cognitive behavioral therapy (CBT) is effective treatment for depression. Many of our patients were suffering from a treatable, but undiagnosed condition. Starting treatment led some patients to postpone or permanently alter their choice for surgery. Others, who had been fearful of a procedure, found they were able to move forward after several weeks of CBT.

While it was clear there were substantial benefits for our patients when they received behavioral services, and we had completed a nice academic study to identify the most sensitive and specific MCS score for hotspotting anxiety and depression, our care delivery process was still failing too frequently. We kept trying to refine the process over many months. Finally, we arrived at a redesign that did work.

Our best solution involved a simple technology tweak. Our patients were completing surveys on laptop computers and their scores were calculated immediately. We wrote a small piece of code that said, "if patient X's MCS score is less than or equal to 35, text behavioral medicine to escort patient X to the exam room" where a behavioral specialist would be ready.

FIGURE 9.3: OPTIMIZED INTEGRATION OF MCS, TECHNOLOGY, AND BEHAVIORAL MEDICINE

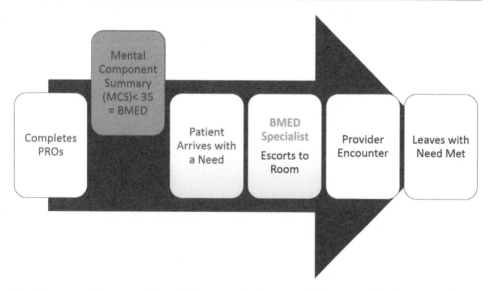

In this way, behavioral medicine specialists could begin a dialogue with the patient about his or her health status measures, including the MCS.

Perhaps the most important lesson learned through the experience was how simple it can be to talk with patients about their mood and mental well-being. After seeing it done dozens of time and then doing it with thousands of patients, it became routine to listen closely as my patient told me about his or her symptoms, and then for me to ask matter-of-factly: "How's your mood been as you deal with all that?" Depending on the patient's response, I'd follow up with, "Would you like any help?"

It can be that simple.

RESOURCES

- » Laderman, M., & Mate, K. (2014) Integrating behavioral health into Primary Care. *Healthcare Executive.* 29(2), 74-77.

- » Collins, C., Hewson D.L., Munger, R., & Wade, T. (2010). *Evolving models of behavioral health integration in primary care.* New York, NY: The Milbank Memorial Fund.

- » Driessen, E., & Hollon, S.D. (2010). *Cognitive behavioral therapy for mood disorders: Efficacy, moderators and mediators.* The Psychiatric Clinics of North America, 33(3), 537–555. doi:10.1016/j.psc.2010.04.005

- » Butler, A.C., Chapman J.E., Forman E.M., & Beck A.T. (2006). The empirical status of cognitive-behavioral therapy: A review of meta-analyses. *Clinical Psychology Review.* 23(1), 17-31.

- » Walsh, T., Hanscom, B., Homa, K., & Abdu, W.A. (2005) The rate and variation of referrals to behavioral medicine services for patients reporting poor mental health in the National Spine Network. *Spine.* 30(6), E154-E160.

- » Walsh, T., Homa, K., Lurie, J., et al. (2006). Detecting depression in patients with chronic spinal pain using the SF-36 health survey. *The Spine Journal.* (6), 16-320.

INTEGRATING SHARED DECISION IN CARE PATHWAYS
WHAT IT IS

When we imagine healthcare, we are likely to think of an astute, compassionate, and brilliant physician listening intently to patients before performing an appropriately targeted physical exam and ordering just the right tests to refute or confirm his diagnosis. The proper diagnosis would then indicate the scientifically proven treatment that should follow. We are even willing to throw out the compassionate part if everything else falls into place, so strong is our desire to be heard and healed.

This is a fairy tale. Like all fairy tales, there are hints of everyday life, but reality is more mundane, and less absolute. The truth is that a concrete diagnosis and a single curative treatment are rare. Scientists estimate that effective care as just described makes up less than 15% of healthcare. The truth is that most diagnoses are somewhat fuzzy, with a margin of error, and treatments have both benefits and potential harms. The situation is complicated further because in the 21st century we are lucky to have multiple treatment options for many diagnoses.

Keeping track of the multiple treatments' risks and benefits is becoming ever more challenging. For example, patients with chronic pain of spinal origin and their providers face decisions regarding:

Possible Treatments for a Patient with Chronic Spine Pain

Medical care
- Anti-inflammatory
- Pain modulating
    - Non-narcotic
    - Narcotic

Injections
- Epidural
- Facet
    - Radiofrequency ablation

Physical Medicine
- Therapy alone
- Therapy in combination with behavioral medicine specialists
- Functional Restoration Program

Surgery
- Decompression
- Fusion
- Augmented fusion
    - Boney
    - Instrumented
    - Anterior
    - Posterior
    - 360

Joint replacements, elective induction for pre-term births, stenting for cardiovascular disease, and hospice care for patients with terminal illness all have multiple treatment options and it is reasonable to believe individual patients, even those with similar physical findings, have individual preferences. Meanwhile, computerized algorithms can help healthcare providers keep the information straight in their own minds, but they are not sufficient. Supporting healthcare providers' decision making falls short in the ability to understand the individual patient.

In 2012, Albert Mulley and colleagues wrote, "Preferences Matter." The authors note that medical training remains solely focused on instructing students to arrive at a correct medical diagnosis. This myopic concentration fails to recognize the explosion in available treatment options and the role of an individual patient's preferences in the treatment decision. The authors define a "preference diagnosis" and describe an urgent need to train healthcare professionals in the skills necessary for making a correct diagnosis of preferences.

More treatment options exist today than ever before, but what is the evidence of a need for additional training? What is the evidence surrounding the diagnosis of patient preferences?

The evidence is plentiful and not flattering. For example, surgical oncologists were asked to estimate the proportion of their patients who would rate "saving my breast" as a top priority regarding their treatment options for breast cancer. On average, the oncologists felt 71% of their patients would rate "saving my breast" very highly. When asked, only 17% of the patients surveyed rated breast conservation as a prime concern. This is a huge misalignment. Now, no study is perfect. There could be something about this particular study that overestimates the difference between physicians' perceptions of what their patients want and what the patients actually say when asked. Imagine for a moment if a similar study was performed again, and the results were 15% better for the physicians, on both sides. The physicians were better able to estimate the truth, and the truth from patients was closer to the physicians' estimate. Such a change in results would be extraordinary (and also extremely unlikely). Regardless, the new results would bring the physicians' estimate down to 56% of patients rating breast conservation as a prime concern and the patients' report up to 32%, hardly erasing the preference misdiagnosis.

In another example, researchers gave de-identified medical records and imaging studies from patients with persistent knee pain to orthopedic surgeons and asked them to point out the cases where replacement of the joint would be an option. The researchers then went to the individuals selected by the surgeons as candidates for the replacement procedure and described all of their treatment. Only 15% of those individuals were interested in an operation at that time. The point here is that there is often a large difference between what healthcare providers consider medically indicated and what patients prefer when they become fully informed of all their options.

Breast cancer and knee pain are not the only conditions with which informed patient preferences weigh heavily. Other researchers, during the late 1990s and early 2000s, found that fully informed, men chose surgical treatment for symptoms of prostate hypertrophy 40% less often than men who had not received complete information; patients with heart disease chose percutaneous interventions 20% less often; patients with one form of spinal condition (disc herniation) chose surgery 30% less often, but patients with another spinal condition (stenosis) chose surgery 30% more often.

The most consistent and important finding from these studies, and the others like them, is that patients make different choices when they are well-informed. Coupled with findings described earlier on the large difference between what patients want and what healthcare providers believe their patients want, even the paternalistic among them can see the need for improving how we inform patients of their options and collaborate with them to arrive at the best decision.

The 3-talk model is a practical approach to engaging patients in deliberations about their healthcare. In its simplest, most easily remembered form, the 3-talk model consists of discussing team formation with your patient, followed by an option talk and then a discussion about his or her decision. These three talks are quite involved, so let's walk through each one.

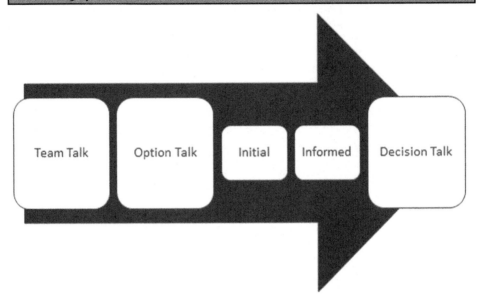

The team talk is where the healthcare professional invites the patient to be part of a team. This is important, because even well-educated, wealthy professionals can be intimidated in a doctor's office or the hospital. They worry their care will suffer if they are not deferential or if they disagree. Real teamwork is not possible in such a setting.

Fortunately, it's fairly easy to create a collaborative environment. You might say something like: "Now that we know what is going on, we need to think about what's next. Fortunately, we have options. While I know the science around the options and I know how my other patients have responded to the different options, you are the expert on what matters most to you. I want to understand what matters most to you, so I need your help. Let's work together; we can make the best decision that will work for you." With that type of communication, the option talk naturally follows.

Here, the healthcare provider will list and describe the options along with the benefits and risks associated with each. If there are gaps in the science, she lets the patient know that the gap is being studied, but, at the moment, there is not yet enough information to know what is best for each person in that area. Pausing between options to check the patient's reactions and answer questions is important. Do they appear tense or uncomfortable? If so, calmly and kindly let the patient know that you have noticed, and ask if they have any questions or concerns before proceeding further.

Writing the options down on a piece of paper as you are having this discussion can be helpful. You want to be sure to cover each option's pluses and the minuses. As healthcare professionals, we have a tendency to emphasize the pluses and minimize the minuses of treatments we prefer, and we need to guard against doing this. Patient decision-support tools can be helpful here. Issue cards, option grids, and decision boards can help during an office visit. Websites and videos can provide information and support beyond the office visit, and can help patients deliberate collaboratively with other important people in their lives.

Summarizing the options and what you have learned about the patient's informed preferences is also vital. Check for understanding at the end of this portion.

In the decision talk, you will make sure the patient's preferences are informed and you'll confirm your understanding of them. Make sure the patient is ready to decide when you reach this step. Sometimes a patient will want to defer a decision, perhaps until they talk to family or another healthcare provider, so ask them, "Are you ready to decide?" or, "Do you want more time?" or, "Are there more things we should discuss?"

If the patient asks, "What would you do?" offer your own thoughts, but remember patients often ask for their healthcare provider's opinion when they are feeling overwhelmed or experiencing decision conflict. Ask what is making this decision so tough for them. If you know them well, it is fine to tentatively say, "Based on what I know about you, it seems like…" Still, be mindful of the ultimate goal—determining what matters most to the individual needing care. Or, consider saying something like, "I hear this is what matters most to you about these options. Am I right about that?"

There you have it. Three little talks—a team talk, an option talk, and a decision talk. They frequently occur within one session, but not always. Sometimes all three have to occur multiple times. Human communication is like that. Remember the model is just to help you understand and refine this new skill set.

And it is a skill to move between the team to the option talk and onto the decision talk, while eliciting preferences in order to figure out what matters most to the patient. Surgeon, writer and public health researcher Atul Gawande described the skill as an evolution from the original paternalistic model of "Dr. Knows Best" to a model where choices are recognized and patients are provided with information. Gawande calls this phase point in the evolution as "Dr. Informative." This is certainly progress from Dr. Knows Best, though many physicians have yet to make it this far in collaborating with their patients. It's often unsettling for patients, and unsatisfying for care providers, to share the more informed physician's role as decision maker with the sick patient. No, "Dr. Informative" is not enough evolution.

Beyond providing information, patient collaboration is critical in eliciting informed preferences going forward and interpreting how those preferences will be integrated into the chosen treatment.

Healthcare providers appear reluctant to adapt the shared decision making model of collaboration, as evidenced by the plethora of academic findings regarding its benefits for patients contrasted with its lack of dissemination. Theories for why shared decision making has not been more widely implemented, such as patients being reluctant to participate and the steps taking too much time and interfering with clinic flow, have been proven to be unfounded. Still another, more cynical, suggestion for why shared decision making has not disseminated includes the potential loss of revenue that could result for surgeons and other proceduralists if patients began declining their treatments *en masse* after watching a video detailing other available options. There is, indeed, some evidence that well-informed patients choose invasive procedures less often than counterparts who have not been fully informed of the risks and benefits of their options. However, the number of studies remains relatively small, and the number of conditions and treatments is also small. The quality of the studies to date are unimpressive, and the effects due to potential biases higher than preferred.

This should also serve as a warning to policy makers and administrators hoping widespread dissemination and implementation of shared decision making will lead to massive societal savings. These savings may materialize, or they may not. As mentioned above, the evidence regarding utilization patterns and savings is nascent. Greater clarity will result with more studies of more conditions using better analytic techniques. The application of some procedures will probably decline but it's just as likely that others will increase. And, in some cases, the procedure may be revisited several times over a decade or more, with the patient choosing more conservative care, until his symptoms or life circumstances change and result in making that procedure inevitable. In such a case, whether researchers find increased or decreased utilization will depend entirely on where they begin and stop measuring.

Policy makers have advocated the use of more straightforward incentives to encourage healthcare providers to complete a shared decision making process with patients. Rather than aiming to curb utilization or cut costs, this simpler approach would involve paying providers who can produce evidence of a collaborative process, or denying payment to those who cannot, and then let the utilization trends fall where they may. This approach, however, has a fatal flaw: There has been no pragmatic way to know whether or not a SDM process has occurred.

In this measurement vacuum, some policy makers and shared decision making advocates have suggested the distribution of tools to help enhance the collaborative process (patient decision support interventions, using academic jargon) could serve as a proxy for the collaborative process. These tools include pamphlets, comparison grids, DVDs, and websites. This is appealing because it is easy to count the number of these tools on a shelf or the clicks on a website at the beginning of a month, the number at the end of the month, and then assume that every tool dispersed or website clicked ensured a collaborative patient-provider encounter.

This line of reasoning appears to be precisely what the writers of the Affordable Care Act had in mind in the run-up to the law's passage. Careful reading of the law reveals how the writers conflated the provision of the tools with the actual process of collaboration.

While this is a wonderful assumption for the creators of decision support interventions, we know it is a false assumption. As pointed out in the three-talk model described earlier, giving patients information about options is a step in the process, but it does not go far enough.

A better measure of collaboration in the clinical encounter would be patient-generated and—reported so it reflected what matters most to patients, not scientists. The measure would be brief and occur immediately following the visit. In addition to being more patient-centered, such an approach would certainly be more pragmatic than recording clinical encounters to be graded later by trained experts. A patient-reported measure of the shared decision making process that was easy to collect and simple to score could also be fed back to providers more quickly, which could improve the training process for the skills necessary for shared decision making skills.

Most healthcare providers receive no training in the skills needed for effective collaboration. The small number who receive training are given lectures on theories regarding communication plus statistical evidence of a mismatch between patient wants and the treatment received. Feedback given to healthcare providers being taught with this approach consists only of test scores from quizzes with questions regarding communication theory and statistics on preference mismatches. That approach is not sufficient for promoting a change in professional behavior. It is entirely possible to achieve a perfect score on a shared decision making quiz, and still do absolutely nothing different during the next patient encounter. Such an approach provides no opportunity to practice new behaviors and there is no feedback to providers regarding their communication skills. Something different is needed.

A better way for training healthcare providers in the skills needed for effective collaboration and shared decision making would involve a brief explanation of the patient's perspective of a good shared decision making process, background on a patient reported measure of the process, and a chance to practice the skills in a safe environment and to receive immediate feedback.

Many organizations now have simulation labs and use trained actors to function as simulated patients. The simulated patients have been used previously to help train healthcare providers in the skills necessary for interviewing a patient, obtaining a verbal history of the patient's health status, and conducting portions of the physical exam. It would also be possible to train the simulated patient to assess the healthcare provider's collaboration skills.

A patient-reported measure that is practical to use would provide the missing link to help policy makers and scientists know when excellent shared decision-making has occurred, as well as what has been needed for a better training method.

CollaboRATE

In order to create a practical patient-reported measure of the shared decision making process, we started by interviewing dozens of patients. What we found surprised us. Patients did not like how we were using the words "decision" and "preferences." They felt decision making in healthcare was different from other cases and they felt talking about preferences in healthcare presented unique circumstances as well. Based on their feedback, we began building a questionnaire and started conducting focus groups of patients to help us build the questions so they made sense to them. After we settled on a set of questions, we went on to test their performance until we had solid evidence the questions were measuring shared decision making, made sense to patients, and performed predictably. We called the patient-reported survey CollaboRATE.

CollaboRATE is a three-item survey that can be texted to patients' cell phones immediately after their healthcare encounter. The three items are:

» How much effort was made to help you understand your health issues?

» How much effort was made to listen to the things that matter most to you about your health issues?

» How much effort was made to include what matters most to you in choosing what to do next?

Each question is graded on a five-point scale from "no effort was made" up to "every effort was made." The entire process takes less than two minutes.

My purpose with this section on shared decision making has been to provide information detailing the need for better collaboration with patients as they consider their treatment options, explain the process of shared decision making, describe a new method for teaching skills necessary for the process to go well, and share a way to assess the process from patients' perspectives. Take a moment to place this in perspective with the other chapters in this book in which I have discussed the use of patient-reported outcomes to document changes in health status and cost allocation to monitor the costs to your organization to produce the goods and services associated with the change in health status. That is the definition of calculating value. Creating a data infrastructure that can do this for every patient enables an organization to then aggregate by patient diagnosis, service line, department, and/or facility.

It is hard to imagine a situation, regardless of the policy environment, where an organization would not thrive if it was able to document high collaboration scores, improvement in patient reported outcomes, and can be transparent about your efforts to control your costs. The organization would be able to "prove" it was delivering care that informed patient chose, improved the health status of patients, all while trying to contain its costs of production.

RESOURCES

» Joosten, E.A.G., DeFuentes-Merillas, L., de Weert, G.H., Sensky, T., van der Staak, C.P.F., & de Jong C.A.J. (2008). Systematic review of the effects of shared decision making on patient satisfaction, treatment adherence, and health status. *Psychother Psychosom*. 77, 219-226.

» Gravel, K., Legare, F., & Graham, I.D. (August 2006) Barriers and facilitators to implementing shared decision making clinical practice: a systematic review of health professionals' perceptions. *Implementation Science*. doi:10.1 186/1748-5908-1-16

» Edwards, A. & Elwyn G. *Shared decision making in health care. Achieving evidence based patient choice*. Oxford University Press. Latest Edition.

» Lee, C.N., Dominik, R., Levin, C.A., Barry, M.J., Cosenza, C., O'Connor, A.M., Mulley, A.G. Jr, & Sepucha, K.R. (2010). Development of instruments to measure the quality of breast cancer treatment decisions. *Health Expectations*. 13(3), 258–72. doi:10.1111/j.1369-7625.2010.00600.x

» Hawker, G.A., Wright, J.G., Coyte, P.C., Williams, J.I., Harvey, B., Glazier, R., Wilkins, A., & Badley, E.M. (2001). 'Determining the need for hip and knee arthroplasty: the role of clinical severity and patients' preferences'. *Medical Care*, 39(3), 206–16

» Frosch, D.L., May, S.G., & Rendle, K.A.S. (May 2012). Authoritarian physicians and patients" fear of being labeled 'difficult' among key obstacles to shared decision making. Health Affairs. 31, 51030-1038

» Elwyn, G., Lloyd, A., May, C., van der Weijden, T., Stiggelbout, A., Edwards, A., Frosch, D.L., Rapley, T., Barr, P.J., Walsh, T., Grande, S.W., Montori, V., & Epstein, R. (2014). Collaborative deliberation: A model for patient care. *Patient Education and Counseling*. 97(2), 158-164.

» Barr, P.J., Thompson, R., Walsh, T., Grande, S.W., Ozanne, E., & Elwyn, G. (2014). The psychometric properties of CollaboRATE. A fast and frugal patient reported measure of shared decision-making process. *J Med Internet Res. 16(1): e2* doi:10.2196/jmir.3085 (Published 14 November 2013)

» Elwyn, G., Barr, P.J., Grande, S.W., Walsh, T., Thompson, R., & Ozanne, E. (2013) Developing CollaboRATE. A fast and frugal measure of shared decision making in clinical encounters. *Patient Educ Couns.* 93(1), 102-7.

» Durand, M.A., Walsh, T., Barr, P.J., Elwyn, G. (2014) Incentiving shared decision making in the USA – Where are we now?" *Healthcare.* Available online November 21, 2014. doi:10.1016/j.hjdsi.2014.10.008

Improving the Patient Experience

Why it is important

Consumer Assessment of Healthcare Providers and Systems (CAHPS) scores are used by Medicare to assess the service quality of healthcare organizations. As we will see, CAHPS scores are an integral part of value-based payment models; however, the primary reasons for wanting to create outstanding experiences for our patients are not financial. The reason we want to create a compassionate, caring experience is because we are caring for humans and for that reason alone. Most of us are all patients at least twice, as we are born and as we die. If you are not transforming healthcare for the patients you currently serve, at least do the work for parents, your children, and yourself. Patients expect convenient access to healthcare and hope for healthcare providers who listen, explain options, and care about their well-being. Patients also expect their healthcare providers to function as a team. They have a basic and reasonable assumption that information provided to one member of the team is retained and made available to all members of the team. CAHPS surveys are an attempt to assess how well we are meeting our patients' hopes and expectations. They sent to patients following their hospital/provider visit and include multiple questions regarding the following seven areas.

1. Getting Timely Care, Appointments, and Information

2. Patient Rating of Doctor

3. Access to Specialist

4. Health Status/Functional Status

5. Shared Decision Making

6. Health Promotion and Education

7. How Well Your Care Providers Communicate

Several conditions and/or treatments are commonly found to be "good places to pilot" improvement projects. These include spine surgeries, hip and knee replacements, the elective induction of preterm births, stenting for blocked arteries of the heart, and concurrent hospice care for patients with a terminal diagnosis. Each of the medical conditions and processes pose difficulties for healthcare administrators and providers working to create reliably excellent patient experiences. Each condition or treatment involves multiple care teams that must communicate and function together over weeks, if not months. Coordinating appointments and sharing data that are critical to the healthcare team and information that matters to patients can be difficult in a single healthcare team. These things become exponentially more difficult as primary-care providers, hospitalists, specialists, nurses and therapists interact over time. Our systems are chaotic and disjointed from the patients' perspective so it is little wonder that CAHPS scores tend to be lower among patients with these diagnoses.

A history of low-quality care, as measured by CAHPS, is a double whammy because these are also high-cost conditions. Value-based contracts include benchmarks for cost reductions as well as provisions for withholding or reducing payments to providers with low CAHPS scores. Insufficient quality scores have been a main reason accountable care organizations fail to obtain the full amount of payments for the savings they were able to achieve for payers. In short, subpar patient experience scores can cost an organization as much as one-fourth of what it would have earned otherwise.

It is not only in the newer payment models where the patient experience affects the bottom line. Evidence reveals that a high level of patient satisfaction is a major driver of long-term financial performance for a healthcare organization in a fee-for-service environment as well, with some estimates suggesting even a 5% dissatisfaction rate among patients can cost a physician $150,000 in revenue over two years from lost patient visits. Meanwhile, the ability to reliably deliver an outstanding experience for patients generates word-of-mouth advertising that has been proven to increase the volume of new patients entering an organization.

FIGURE 9.5: THE SEVEN DOMAINS OF CAHPS MEASURES

MICROSYSTEM FUNCTION
1. Getting Timely Care, Appointments, and Information
2. Patient Rating of Doctor
3. Access to Specialist
PATIENT GENERATED AND REPORTED HEALTH STATUS
4. Health Status / Functional Status
SHARED DECISION MAKING
5. Shared Decision Making
6. Health Promotion and Education
7. How Well Your Care Providers Communicate

The clinical microsystem is where healthcare is delivered and process mapping from the patient's perspective is the key to understanding issues of timeliness, patient-provider communication, and access. The microsystem is also where shared decision making occurs. Health promotion and education are frequently aspects of the option talk described in the shared decision making chapter. Assessing the patient's health and functional status is best done with patient generated measures as described in the prior chapter on measurement. What has been missing so far is a discussion of how microsystems thinking, patient-reported measures, and shared decision making can work harmoniously to help improve communication within and between provider teams.

Healthcare providers work in teams, but communication among members of a healthcare team, especially members with different background training and unique professional languages, can be challenging. The first thing to realize about team communication is that the team comprises individuals each with a relationship with every other team member, and as in every relationship, the relationships with the team members will suffer if they are not attended to. Across many practice types, physicians tend to work independently, frequently moving from a clinic setting, to a hospital setting, and to sometimes a surgical setting. At each location, other care team members work to coordinate interaction between a physician and her patients. It can be difficult for care teams to welcome rotating physicians one after the other, each with his or her own idiosyncrasies. Each setting also has its own communication styles, workflow and workarounds. This type of work dynamic can be challenging to both physicians and other workers alike. Moving from one care team to another, without truly knowing the inner workings of a particular team, is challenging and one of the greatest difficulties is ensuring the integration of a particular patient's informed preferences.

A healthcare provider who understands the shared decision making process will have made every effort to explain the options that exist, and support the patient as he moves from naïve choices toward informed preferences. He will make every effort to elicit those informed preferences from the patient and then to integrate them into the patient's treatment plan. Process mapping a patient's journey through a microsystem can identify places and tasks where the team's focus strays from what matters most to the patient. Using the CollaboRATE survey can help assess how well the team is staying focused and monitor improvement efforts.

A single provider attempting to improve the patient experience will soon find her efforts stymied if she cannot communicate the patient's informed preferences to other team members. It is challenging because providers often feel isolated and aren't aware that they are part of multiple teams. Providers become frustrated when they have given orders to one team only to find another team ignorant of it. Worse still, while team members worry about fitting in and adapting to different physician demands, patients can remain isolated, frustrated, sick, and vulnerable. Many patients have claimed that they feel like their provider knows his diagnosis but doesn't really "get" him as a person. We are all frustrated by the lack of integration, and patients suffer for it.

Relational coordination expert Jody Hoffer Gittell and colleagues have examined when relationships and communication are most likely to be strained within a team. They have found higher levels of strained relationships and communication breakdown when necessary tasks require interdependence, must be done quickly, and have a lot of variability, uncertainty, and multiple options. Interdependence, variability, uncertainty, multiple options, and time constraints describe everyday life in the healthcare industry. Good relationships and good communication can act as antidotes. They increase our capacity for processing information and provide social support. If the members of a microsystem all know and have shared the patient's goals for a successful outcome, stress is lessened for the microsystem and the patient, and responsibilities and tasks are more easily identified and completed.

How these changes occur within a team has also been the subject of research by Gittell and her colleagues. They have found coordination among members of a team improves when team members share goals and knowledge, and have mutual respect for one another. All these aspects are only conveyed through communication. We know that team members assess their microsystem's function more favorably when communication among members occurs regularly, that relevant information is shared or made available when it is most needed, that the information is accurate, and that it is focused on completing the task at hand. Communication suffers, in contrast, when it is infrequent, delayed, based on assumptions irrespective of accuracy, and focused on placing blame over finding solutions. These features of good relationships and good communication are basic and interrelated, but frequently left unconsidered among members of clinical microsystems.

Building good relationships within a microsystem takes conscious effort. And the best way to begin starts with improving the communication between a healthcare provider and a patient. The process of shared decision making creates a healthcare provider with deep knowledge of a patients' informed preferences and goals. Sharing this knowledge of the patient's goals—and preferences for achieving them—helps to establish better care coordination and ensures that "what matters most" to the patient is integrated into the care plan.

Healthcare has become more complex, with patients are frequently cared for by multiple teams, which requires information about the patient to be transferred from one microsystem to another. The handoff is the transfer of patient information, along with professional responsibility and accountability for the patient, between individuals and teams. Some of these handoffs occur within professions (primary care to specialist to hospitalist to primary care) and some among professions (doctor to nurse to physical therapist to social worker).

Handoffs are a vulnerable time for patients. There is no standardized way to conduct a handoff, so methods differ from one setting to another. There are, however, features of excellent coordination and communication between healthcare teams. Whenever possible, a handoff should happen in person. This is not always possible, so it is even more important for the current care provider to first compose his or her thoughts. Of course, you will also include medical information, but this should also be a time when you share your preference diagnosis. Describing the options that have been discussed with the patient as well as the patient's preferences about those options is important. This knowledge of the patient as a person with the medical condition, not just as a diagnostic code, is what makes care truly patient-centered and integrated within and among clinical microsystems.

IntegRATE

Many patients describe their healthcare experiences as chaotic, confusing and personally cold. They would prefer healthcare professionals who care for them as unique humans and work in well-integrated teams. In the previous section on shared decision making, I suggested that the shared decision-making process is a skill set that can be learned and, when performed well, improves communication between healthcare providers and patients. The skills can be assessed and progress can be monitored using the CollaboRATE patient survey. In this chapter, I have outlined how well-done shared decision making produces knowledge of what matters most to a patient, and how communicating this knowledge within a microsystem and among microsystems can lead to more integrated care. But, how would we know if care was truly more integrated?

A review of the current measures of care integration and continuity found no consensus, even regarding the basic concept of integration, among the various measures examined. The most notable and consistent finding was the lack of patients' perspectives in the construction of the measurement tools. After the exhaustive review, a top-down approach to assessing care continuity was recommended to be, if not abandoned, at least supplemented by an assessment that captured how patients perceive the integration of their care. This led researchers at Dartmouth College to re-assess the topic, using techniques that have been proven to work well for constructing patient-generated and -reported measures. As described in the chapters on outcome measures and shared decision making, this approach begins with multiple patient interviews in which the scientists share a medical or scientific concept with subjects, then seek to understand how the concept is perceived by the subject, and then create language that expresses the subject's perception. Over the course of multiple interviews, some expressions recur much more than others. The recurrent expressions are then tested with groups of subjects in a focus group setting. Over multiple focus groups, a single expression is found that best captures the original concept as understood by patients.

Using these techniques, the Dartmouth researchers were able to identify four features that patients use to identify highly integrated healthcare. The features were: effective sharing of personal and health information, consistency with explanations and advice, witnessing respect and collaboration among the healthcare team members, and clarity regarding the roles of each member of the microsystem. Questions were developed using these four features in order to help patients assess their care integration.

TABLE 9.1: FEATURES OF INTEGRATED CARE AND QUESTIONS TO ASSESS

Features of integrated care as defined by patients	Assessment survey questions
Information Sharing	How often did you have to do or explain something because people did not share information with each other?
Consistent Advice	How often were you confused because people gave you conflicting information or advice?
Mutual Respect	How often did you feel uncomfortable because people did not get along with each other?
Role Clarity	How often were you unclear whose job it was to deal with a specific question or concern?

This chapter has covered the importance ensuring patients experience a tightly integrated and patient-centered healthcare system. This aspect of value has frequently been unaddressed and the lack of attention has caused healthcare providers to lose out on reimbursements they have otherwise earned. More important than the financial impact, integrated, patient-centered care is what we want for our parents and children. Medicare attempts to measure the patient experience using CAHPS scores that they collect with lengthy surveys.

The results of the surveys are fed back to providers and systems weeks, and sometimes months, after the fact. Organizations wanting to improve the patient experience should focus on improving relationships within and among their own microsystems by focusing on better communication and better handoffs. The skills needed to achieve high levels of coordination and excellent handoffs begin with the shared decision-making process between a patient and a provider. These skills are trainable. Current abilities and the effects of training can be assessed using CollaboRATE. Additional skills are needed at the team level where sharing goals and knowledge in a respectful manner come to the fore. Communicating goals and knowledge in a timely manner, honestly and accurately, and staying focused on integrating patients' preferences all help to improve coordination within a microsystem. A mindful approach to the handoff process between microsystems helps to ensure the integration of care across microsystems.

RESOURCES

» Drain, M., & Kaldenberg, D.O. (1999). Building patient loyalty and trust: The role of patient satisfaction. *Group Practice Journal*. 1999. 48(9), 32-35.

» Rubin, H.R., et al. (1993) Patients' ratings of outpatient visits in different practice settings: Results from the Medical Outcomes Study." *JAMA.*. 270(7), 835-840.)

» Elwyn G., Barr, P.J., & Walsh, T et al. (2013). Developing CollaobRATE: A fast and frugal patient-reported measure of shared decision making. Patient Education and Counseling. 93, 102-107

» McEvoy, P., Escott, D., & Bee, P (2011). Case Management for high-intensity service users: toward a relational approach to care coordination. *Health and Social Care in the Community*. 19(1) 60 – 69.

» Gittell, J.H., Fairfield K.M., Bierbaum, B., Head, W., Jackson, R., Kelly, M., Laskin, R., Lipson, S., Siliski J., Thornhill, T., & Zuckerman, J. (2000). Impact of Relational Coordination on Quality of Care, Postoperative Pain and Functioning and Length of Stay: A Nine-Hospital Study of Surgical Patients. *Medical Care*. 38(8), 807-819.

» Uijen, A.A., Heinst, C.W., Schellevis, F.G., van den Bosch, W.J.H.M., van de Laar, F.A., Terwee, C.B., et al. (2012). Measurement properties of questionnaires measuring continuity of care: a systematic review. PLoS One. 7(7), e42256

» Uijen, A.A., Schers, H.J., van Weel, C. (2013) Continuity of care preferably measured from the patients' perspective. *Journal of Clinical Epidemiology.* 63(9), 998–9.

» Singer, S.J., Burgers, J., Friedberg, M, Rosenthal, M.B., Leape, L., & Schneider, E. (2011) Defining and measuring integrated patient care: promoting the next frontier in health care delivery. *Medical Care Research and Review.* 68(1):112–27.

» Elwyn, G., Thompson, R., John, R., & Grande, S. (March 2015) Developing IntegRATE: a fast and frugal patient-reported measure of integration in healthcare delivery. *Int J Integr Care.* 15.

» Ham, C. (2010). The ten characteristics of the high-performing chronic care system. *Health Economics, Policy and Law.* 2010. 5(1), 71–90.

LEARNING COLLABORATIVE

Continual improvement is enhanced when multiple clinics join together in a collaborative dedicated to improving the value of care delivered. In this chapter I will describe several examples of successful learning collaboratives and how they have used the principles and techniques outlined in this book to foster their success.

THE NATIONAL SPINE NETWORK

http://www.nationalspinenetwork.org

The NSN was formed in 1994 by several large research-oriented practices in order to facilitate data collection during multi-centered research. Members of the NSN pioneered the use of patient-reported outcomes for clinical research. In the earliest days of the collaborative, patients were completing paper-based surveys that were then entered into a spreadsheet by research assistants. By 2000, the network was using tablet-based data entry by patients immediately before their clinical encounter. Clinicians at the Dartmouth-Hitchcock Spine Center began a practice of printing the patient's survey in order to review the document *with the patient at the point of service.*

Over time, the process has been refined further to allow patients to complete their data entry online and for the information to be uploaded to the patient's record and available for review by the clinician before the clinic encounter. This novel approach to the use of "outcome" data led to numerous insights, including the integration of behavioral medicine specialists within the clinic microsystem described previously. This increased integration with behavioral medicine, and decreased numbers of non-surgical candidates appearing on surgeon's clinic schedules.

The NSN is a non-profit organization with a mission to improve the quality of care for patients with pain and loss of function due to spine problems, improve the productivity of providers caring for these patients, and improve research cost-effectiveness by streamlining relevant data collection to patients. Joining the network and purchasing the customizable software allows new members to quickly begin using patient-reported measures, integrates those measures into existing health records, allows comparisons between a clinic and the NSN as a whole, as well as comparisons between multiple providers within a clinic. By their own estimates, the software saves a practice as much as $30,000 per clinician per year through reduced administrative overhead, the elimination of dictation and transcription, and improved billing compliance. More importantly, the use of patient-reported data can be used to improve knowledge of what works, and why, for patients at your organization as well as enhancing your ability to detect comorbid conditions.

THE CALIFORNIA JOINT REPLACEMENT REGISTRY

http://www.caljrr.org

The CJRR began in 2009 as a combined effort between the California Healthcare Foundation, the Pacific Business Group on Health, and the California Orthopedic Association. With 47 hospitals participating, the CJRR registry is "Level III," meaning it collects and incorporates clinical and patient-reported information for quality improvement. The registry publishes, for willing providers, patient-reported outcomes by hospital in order to identify best-practices and to help members identify and prioritize areas for improvement efforts. The table below comes from the CJRR website and shows the response rate for six participating facilities as well as the proportion of patients reporting meaningful improvement.

PERCENT OF PATIENTS THAT REPORTED A MEANINGFUL IMPROVEMENT IN THEIR PHYSICAL ABILITIES AFTER HIP AND KNEE JOINT REPLACEMENT SURGERY, BY HOSPITAL

Hospital	Total Surgical Patients	Completed Survey	Response %	% Patients with Meaningful Improvement
A	793	554	69	88
B	327	66	20	87
C	3078	199	7	87
D	128	45	35	87
E	224	42	19	86
F	499	72	14	83

Interestingly, the percentage of patients improving is similarly high across all hospitals. Now imagine that this table contained two more columns— one for the estimated costs and another for average reimbursement. These data do not have to be publicly reported, but they could be shared between selected colleagues. The American Joint Replacement Institute will have over 450 participating hospitals. It would be possible to create small learning groups composed of similar hospitals, but from different geographic regions so no competing hospitals were grouped together. Such an approach would make for a strong learning collaborative.

At the time of its inception, CJRR members are recognized by agreement as quality-focused providers by Anthem, Blue Shield, Covered California, UnitedHealthcare, and other health insurance organizations. As of March 31, 2015, the CJRR transitioned to the American Joint Replacement Registry. This will increase the size of the registry by a factor of ten. While the process is ongoing, the aim is to bring all the same benefits to participants across the country. The work done by this registry helps to demonstrate another benefit of adapting patient-reported outcomes: Payers recognize their use as signal of provider quality and commitment to continuous improvement.

THE NORTHERN NEW ENGLAND CARDIOVASCULAR DISEASE STUDY GROUP

http://www.nnecdsg.org/about.htm

The NNECDSG began in 1987 in order to address variation in the rates for coronary artery bypass grafts, percutaneous coronary intervention, and heart valve replacement. From the beginning the founders have met monthly or quarterly to review the various rates from across the region, build shared knowledge and language, and most importantly, build trust. Over several such meetings, it became clear to all that the variation in rates could not be explained by illness severity, poverty, race, or education. The regional facilities were too much alike in those regards while the procedural rates varied widely. Slowly, consensus grew around the concept of shared decision making with patients as the group realized that determining the right rate required an assessment of the patients' medical need and an assessment of each patient's preferences regarding the risk and benefits of each treatment option.

The founders created a registry, similar to the approach outlined in the sections above, and then went further with their regular meetings and discussions of shared decision making. One of the first group projects was to build decision support tools for the cardiology teams. This multistep process began with the group collectively reviewing the published evidence and coming to consensus regarding the clinical indicators for each procedure. Then a customized informed consent procedure was created, tested, modified and finally implemented across the group.

The informed consent process varied widely from one organization to another. Some did not describe procedural options, quantify risks, or give alternatives. Modifying the informed consent process to include more information about options, along with the risks and benefits of each, started a shared decision-making process with patients that has eventually led to an interactive predictive statistical model that clinicians use to help patients understand their risks. In this way, the NNECDSG created the first combined patient and provider decision-support tool to facilitate a shared decision-making process. This resulted in the organizational rates for coronary artery bypass grafts drifting more toward the average rate of the group as a whole, that is, variation was reduced.

Over time, the registry data produced insights, educating the organizations rapidly and further spreading the best practices model. For example, complications with kidney function were found to vary across the network from as little as 2.3% of patients to a high of 6.6%. The contrast agent used to visualize coronary vessels it was discovered could damage kidneys. Seeing this, the group used the same methods that had helped reduce variation in bypass procedures to adjust for this issue.

The initial step consisted of collectively reviewing the medical literature for best practices and gaining consensus for an approach to improving care. The group considered the sites with the lowest complication rates to be benchmarks they would all strive to achieve. The improvement plan was then implemented across the group membership, except for the benchmark sites and two additional organizations serving as controls. The intervention worked. Complication rates decreased at the intervention sites, but no change was seen at the benchmark or control sites. Seeing the improvement, all organizations followed and complication rates were reduced at the control sites and even the benchmark sites. Overall, the rate of kidney damage from the contrast agent declined 21%, and 28% for the highest-risk patients.

THE OHIO PERINATAL QUALITY COLLABORATIVE

https://www.opqc.net

The OPQC is a statewide collaborative of perinatal clinics committed to using quality improvement principles to reduce early elective inductions, reduce pre-term births, and improve birth outcomes for women and infants. To achieve these goals, the group collaboratively reviewed evidence-based protocols and built consensus within the group where evidence was sparse. The agreed-upon evidence was disseminated to all clinics. Patient information packets were produced and disseminated in a similar manner.

The group's first project focused on understanding the statewide variation in early inductions that are either necessary or elective procedures. The first step was to build the capacity to differentiate the two. Among participating organizations, the rate of early elective inductions varied from 5% to15%. This was troubling because, as one group member stated, "The reasons for early elective induction are not well-documented, but the risks to the infant are." The increased risks can lead to increased lengths of stay in hospitals, admissions to neonatal intensive care, and greater costs to families and payers, all resulting from a procedure that, by definition, is not necessary.

Group members received the decision-support tools and attended workshops sponsored by OPQC. In return, the member organizations were expected to:

> » Provide senior leadership who would serve as contact points and project sponsors
>
> » Provide resources for team members to work on preparation for workshops, conference calls, as well as the development and testing of change efforts
>
> » Send three obstetrics team members to the workshops
>
> » Perform pre-work to prep for the workshops
>
> » Participate in monthly conference calls
>
> » Connect the goals of OPQC to their home organization
>
> » Use standard data-collection tools
>
> » Keep and share measures and experiences through monthly reports

The demanding approach worked. Among the 20 participating sites, early elective inductions declined from over 15% in 2008 to less than 5% in 2010. The OPQC's efforts extended beyond their collaborative, evidenced by a statewide decline from an average of roughly 13% to between 7% and 8%. For Ohio, this equates to approximately 6,000 births going to full term and a decline of approximately 180 neonatal intensive care unit admissions *per year.*

The Leapfrog Group has reported a dramatic decline in early elective inductions nationwide. Across the United States in 2010, an average of 17% of births were early elective inductions and by 2013 the average had declined to 4.6%. These results among organizations reporting data are impressive, and the number of participating organizations continues to rise. However, as seen in Leapfrog's own data, most organizations do not yet participate or decline to publically report their data. Even among organizations choosing to report, rates in the 20% to 30+% range remain.

The question then is, "What is your organization's rate of early elective inductions?" Knowing the answer and working to lower the rate below 5% if necessary provides insights regarding how to use improvement methods, improve an infant's and mother's health, lower costs, reduce the amount billed to patients and payers, and how to implement or participate in a learning collaborative. The experience provides an early, quick "win" on this important work, and can help build momentum for further efforts throughout an organization.

THE CYSTIC FIBROSIS FOUNDATION

http://www.cff.org/treatments/CFCareGuidelines

The Cystic Fibrosis (CF) Foundation began developing its registry and patient-centered approach 50 years ago. At the time, most children diagnosed with CF did not attend elementary school and died by their early teens. Now, the average life expectancy is in the mid-40s. Much of this improvement is due to advances in the how families and patients have learned to care for themselves.

The registry consists of 110 centers reporting data on a patient's lung function and nutritional status. In addition, close attention is paid to the percentage of CF sufferers screened for CF-related diabetes as well as the percent of CF sufferers with recommended visit cycles. Too few or too many visits can be signs of trouble that need to be explored, so organizations use a reminder system to alert them when variations from the recommend cycle occur and staff reach out to the patients in order to determine the root cause.

The annual data from the registry are summarized and made available to all organizations, providers and patients in a yearly report. Lessons learned are collected, and inform a quality improvement toolkit created for patients and families. The toolkit includes tips for succeeding and inspiration for patients "from people like you." Patients and families are taught to be proactive about their needs. They are taught to ask, "What can I do to take better care of myself?" and "What would ideal care be for me?" Patients are also queried to find out what works well at their centers and what could help them receive better care from their providers. Responses are tabulated and discussed across the network. Fifty years on, and with over a hundred organizations, completely new concerns are rare. This means an answer is likely available from somewhere in the collaborative whenever an organization experiences an unforeseen hardship.

THE CENTER TO ADVANCE PALLIATIVE CARE

https://www.capc.org

Research has shown that most patients, fully informed of their conditions and the risks and benefits of their treatment options, choose to die at home with their family and without heroic life-extending measures. Many of these patients express this preference verbally and in writing. Still, over 50% of patients end up dying in an ICU, intubated and unable to communicate. The CAPC began in 2008 in order to promote standardization and improve the quality of care delivered to patients with a terminal illness. There is no charge to an organization for joining CAPC, providing data, or for receiving a report. The registry includes variables on the structure and process of palliative care, including the service model, department size and composition, hours of available service, the number of consultations/admissions, as well as the average patient age, race, and ethnicity, the most common diseases, origin of the request for consultation, the total number of hospital deaths, average length of stay, and total number of beds at the organizations. These data are then organized into four categories: operational, clinical, customer, and financial.

Understanding the care-giving structure and process at participating organizations, it is hoped, can help determine why and how patients' expressed preferences are so frequently overridden. Some evidence suggests that poorly integrated care is a major contributor to the problem. Researchers at Dartmouth have developed the hospital care intensity index, which measures the number of days patients spend in the hospital and the number of physician visits the patients were exposed to during the last six months of life. Another variable measures the proportion of patients cared for by 10 or more physicians. More days in hospital, more visits and more doctors all work to increase the intensity and make it more difficult to coordinate care. Regions with lower-intensity care do not suffer from shorter life expectancy or less satisfied patients or families. Indeed, the opposite appears true. Regions with fewer hospital days and fewer doctor visits use hospice and palliative care services at higher rates. These services have been shown to lessen pain and depressive symptoms, and increase patient and family satisfaction. Some data suggest the less intense approach prolongs life.

One difficulty with trying to lessen the intensity of care is that a major driver of high intensity is simply the number of intensive care beds in a region containing multiple hospitals. To understand this phenomenon, disregard the ICU and look instead hospital patient admittance decisions. Consider two identical patients, both equally ill and with similar family support. Both are sick enough that admission to the hospital is being considered, but is not emergent. If a hospital bed is available, the patient will be admitted. If all hospital beds are full, the patient's medications can be adjusted, nurses can visit his home the following day, and a follow-up visit in the clinic will be scheduled for a few days' time. Regions with more hospital beds per 1,000 Medicare beneficiaries admit patients like this much more frequently than hospitals with fewer beds. This has nothing to do with how sick the patient is—it is merely a function of the available supply of beds. Admission to intensive care is similarly sensitive to the supply of regional resources. This is not a fault of the care providers. Indeed, they cannot see the effect being exerted by the total number of beds in a region (not just their own facility). Simply put, the supply of resources exerts a pressure that induces greater care intensity, and greater intensity can lead to poorly coordinated care that can swamp the expressed wishes of patients. Moreover, the providers have no measurable means for pushing back. They cannot close beds on their own accord, and leaving beds unused in a fee-for-service environment leads to an administrative reprimand.

The patient-reported assessment tool, IntegRATE, may be able to help. The tool is currently under development; and its reliability and validity have yet to be established, but it's meant to address just this kind of issue. The promise of a patient-reported measure of shared decision making (CollaboRATE) and the continuity of care (IntegRATE) lies in their ability to quickly provide actionable feedback to care providers.

CHAPTER 10

PUTTING IT ALL TOGETHER

Patient-centered outcomes are vital to the success of any healthcare organization. Knowledge of the patient as a person with the medical condition is how we create truly patient-centered and integrated care. These are not arcane concepts. Outcomes of value to patients, accountants, hospital administrators, legal counsel, board members, and providers alike are fairly basic and easily grasped—like health status, and a patient's ability to function, for example.

The 20th century moral and political philosopher John Rawls often asked his students to imagine designing a society from the ground up—government, healthcare, education, everything.

I like to modify that concept and have my students imagine designing a healthcare system from scratch. Who's going to deliver which types of care? Who is going to pay for it?

That's a very powerful position to be in, but I tell them the price of having all that power is that you and your family will have to use the system you design with no knowledge of how you would enter that system. You don't know whether you're going to be healthy and of sound mind or sick or mentally challenged. You don't know whether you're going to be rich or poor, or black or white. How would that affect how you design it?

I ask my students after they've considered that question whether any of them would design a system the way ours exists today. Of course, given that scenario, nobody would.

A tension exists between system we would want and the system we have. My response to that tension is to work to fix that. It's an ethical imperative to take steps to make the healthcare system that I'm part of more like the system I would design for myself and my family.

The situation is not that hypothetical. You don't know what your healthcare needs are going to be. You don't know whether you're going to be hit by a bus, or if your child is going to have seizures, or if one of your parents is going to develop a debilitating chronic disease.

We need to be working on creating a better healthcare system now.

You may be satisfied with your organization's operation and your patients' satisfaction with the care you provide them, so you might ask, "Why should I do anything different now?"

The simple answer is that the world is changing, whether we like it or not. It's changing rapidly and will affect your volume of patients, your hospital's or practice's finances, and the quality of care you provide. The major drivers of these changes are the pressure to slow the growth of healthcare spending and to reform how it is paid for, including new payment schemes that move away from volume to value, and new methods for measuring the quality of care.

We need to be working on this now because the changes will affect your livelihood, but just as importantly, you, your child, and your parents will one day need the system we create.

RISING HEALTHCARE COSTS BECOME AN INCREASING DRAG ON RESOURCES

Rising healthcare spending caused by inefficiencies in the system is a drag on resources available for education, infrastructure, emergency response, and many other necessary services.

Healthcare spending has slowed recently for a variety of reasons, including the economy and the Affordable Care Act. There is a legitimate debate there. However, no one is arguing whether healthcare spending will continue upward. The Centers for Medicare and Medicaid Services have estimated that by 2021 healthcare spending is expected to reach 20% of our GDP. Perhaps more worrisome, by that year, healthcare will be the largest driver of our national debt for the foreseeable future.

The situation is dire locally. State and local governments are struggling to pay for healthcare. These expenditures include not only covering Medicaid, but also insurance premiums, and needed care, for state workers, including police, fire service, road crews and teachers, among others. Healthcare expenditures are eating up state funds that could be made available for safety, infrastructure and education.

I have informally talked with leaders in several small towns and municipalities and asked them what keeps them up at night, and they often answer that it is healthcare and the expense of providing it to the people who keep the lights on, fix the roads and make things run smoothly. All it takes is one of those employees with one very sick family member to cause an insurer to modify the rate for everyone, causing premiums to rise even as much as 25 to 30 percent in a bad year.

Mayors, town managers or city council members cannot do their yearly budgets for everything else without knowing what that premium is going to be. The same thing can be said for many health system and medical group management executives.

EVOLVING PAYMENT SCHEMES BRING GREATER RISK AND RESPONSIBILITY

As mentioned early in the first chapter, healthcare payment reform is nearly constant and change will continue, such as seen with the unfolding of Value-Based Payments to hospital systems and the Medicare Access and CHIP Reauthorization Act and its Merit-based Incentive Payment System (MIPS). Again, knowing what matters most to patients, and trying to improve those outcomes, while maintaining or lowering the costs to achieve those outcomes, will create greater value regardless of political winds.

New payment schemes have moved away from fee for service, which tended to incentivize an ever greater volume of care while placing the risk of unnecessary or low-quality care solely on the payer. These new payments move toward methods that place a financial risk onto healthcare provider networks and link payments to the quality of care delivered and outcomes achieved.

FEE FOR SERVICE

The financial exposure in fee-for-service systems is on payers, who risk paying for unnecessary or low quality care.

FEE FOR SERVICE	
Description	Payment regardless of outcome, quality or efficiency
Financial Risk	Payer only
Where in Medicare (2015)	Less than 15%

PAY FOR PERFORMANCE

Pay for performance is an attempt to link payment to quality. It is still based on fee for service—as long as quality and outcome benchmarks are met. This payment strategy is meant to reward providers for higher quality necessary care.

PAY FOR PERFORMANCE	
Description	A portion of payment is based on outcome, quality and/or efficiency
Financial Risk	Shared
Where in Medicare (2015)	Less than 15%

BUNDLED PAYMENTS

Bundled episodes are payments to providers and health systems that consist of a single payment meant to cover the cost of care by multiple providers over a defined period as long as quality benchmarks are met. An "episode" might consist of the three days prior to and 30 days following a knee replacement surgery, or a year's worth of diabetes care. Fee for service continues for all other care. This method is meant to make the payment for high-cost/high-volume care more predictable and to decrease the payers' risk of paying for unnecessary care or low-quality care. As in the pay-for-performance method, providers who cannot demonstrate excellent outcomes and high-quality care will be paid less than providers who can.

Bundles also place a new financial exposure on providers—that the risk of necessary care that exceeds the bundled amount. This is an attempt to balance risk between payers and providers.

BUNDLED PAYMENTS	
Description	A portion of payment is capped for certain diagnoses and timeframes, remainder still based on volume with outcome, quality and efficiency benchmarks
Financial Risk	Shared
Where in Medicare (2015)	Financially and clinically integrated networks, Accountable Care Organizations, Medical homes

SHARED SAVINGS

Shared savings is a payment strategy where networked providers are rewarded with a percentage of any net savings that result from their efforts to reduce healthcare spending for a target population, as long as outcome and quality benchmarks are met. This further reduces the payer's risk of over-payment and creates a new incentive for providers to practice as efficiently as possible while maintaining excellent outcomes and high quality. It is a method that involves shared risks and shared rewards.

SHARED SAVINGS	
Description	Providers are offered a percentage of net savings from efforts to reduce spending for a target population
Financial Risk	Shared
Where in Medicare (2015)	Financially and clinically integrated networks, Accountable Care Organizations, Medical homes

CAPITATION

Capitation consists of a global payment to a network of providers for each of their patients, as long as outcome and quality criteria are met, regardless of diagnosis or episode. Providers remain exposed to the risk of necessary care exceeding the negotiated payment amount.

CAPITATION	
Description	Providers are accountable for the quality and efficiency of care for patients over long periods of time
Financial Risk	Shared
Where in Medicare (2015)	Established clinically integrated networks (e.g., Pioneer Accountable Care Organizations)

Taken together, pay for performance, bundles, shared savings, and capitation are considered "alternative payments." Bundles, shared savings, and capitation are also considered risk-based. Alternative payments are growing rapidly.

Risk-based models are preferred by all payers, not just Medicare, because they reduce their risk of paying for unnecessary or low-quality care and they make their expenses more predictable. Commercial payers, therefore, wish to follow Medicare's lead.

NEW METHODS FOR MEASURING QUALITY OF CARE

There is no arguing that improving patient outcomes requires data, but rather than getting lost in big data processes and systems, providers need to focus on *data that matters most.*

Quality measures are typically payer- or provider-centric. Did the provider get the technical details correct? Were the standards followed?

Outcome measures are different. They can be provider-centric, (e.g., did the spinal fusion procedure achieve intersegmental fusion?) or patient-centric, such as mortality, pain, health status and function. These can be collected by both providers and payers.

There are several methods payers may use to assess patient care quality. First, payers may use billing data. Screening rates and medication usage that compare your practice to a larger network or the nation are typical examples of these measures. Substantial problems can occur with this approach, however. These include the fact that data from a small practice of several doctors may not represent your organization, organization-wide data may not represent individual providers within the system, and sample sizes at the individual provider-level can become very small when other relevant variables are taken into account. When combined, these limitations can make obscure meaningful findings—enough to lead to either corrective action or efforts to disseminate positive findings.

Payers can also assess quality using patient surveys. In addition to the previously mentioned problems with meaningfulness, aggregation, and sample size, patient surveys—as they are currently conducted by payers—ask patients to recall visits that occurred weeks or even months past. Response rates to these surveys are typically very low and tend to reflect a patient's health status and sense of well-being during the time of the survey, not the time of the actual visit.

The best patient reported measures are built from patient-generated projects. That is, patients have told us, "These things matter to us and should be measured/monitored." We, as scientists, then build the measure for patients to use. The creation of the CollaboRATE measure to assess the process of shared decision making is a great example of this type of work.

The CollaboRATE model asks patients to evaluate how much effort you put into helping them understand their health issues, how well you listened to the things that mattered most to them about their health issues, and then how well you and your team followed through in communicating and including their preferences in their care.

Patient preferences matter. Shared decision making matters.

SELLING VALUE TO THE DECISION MAKERS

Committed individuals in healthcare delivery organizations around the country are working to make the shift from volume- to value-based payment arrangements. While a few pioneering health systems are well into the transition, most organizations are not and remain anxious about any future transition. New legislation gets phased in over multiple years spanning election cycles that contain vague political promises to revert back to previous payment systems or implement newer, as yet unspecified, changes. It is a chaotic, uncertain landscape.

The leaders are anxious because they are "navigating blind." They lack essential data on outcomes that matter to patients and the costs associated with achieving those outcomes. Where data already exist, they do not know how to find, retrieve and organize it. Perhaps most importantly, they do not know how to leverage data to chart the best path forward.

Meanwhile, a booming "big data" industry complicates the situation with promises to solve an organization's data needs through the addition of costly infrastructure. The electronic records and servers produce voluminous data that can quickly smother an organization with useless and confusing numbers if the leaders do not have a plan for turning the data to action.

Big data alone is not enough. We need to focus on finding existing data and creating systems to capture information that matters. And we must create systems and processes that help to leverage data and propel an organization's transition to value-based care.

Any transformation effort comes with costs. A significant challenge quality leaders face is communicating the necessity for creating true value to the people in their organizations who have the power to actualize it. That means the people who are your top decision makers need to literally "buy in" to your organization's improvement projects—people like board members, department chiefs, and senior administrators.

Surveys have found that less than a third of hospital boards have received any formal training in healthcare delivery and quality improvement, and only a fifth of organizations reported that the chairperson, or the board or one of its committees was an influential force for improving quality throughout their hospitals. Too few of these top decision makers are aware of how their organizations compare in the quality of healthcare delivery with their competitors or with national benchmarks.

A tendency exists amongst various kinds of academics to assume that everything we discuss is well known and understood, this is partly because we're speaking in an echo chamber and hearing the same things over and over again, and because we tend to talk to only a few people (who also tend to be like us). We write to impress our peers, not to disseminate widely. While this is understandable in a publication model that relies on peer-review, it is clear, when we leave our campuses and get out in other places, that not everything we know trickles down stream, and a lot of work remains to be done.

To get the buy-in of the board, your team must demonstrate which of its innovations has the potential to lead to meaningful improvement and they need to explain it in terms that make sense to people who may not understand the finer points of managing healthcare delivery. The board and top executive leadership leaders need to understand why optimizing value needs to be a top priority, and they need to know that only positive, substantial changes that are meaningful to patients or the team constitute true improvement.

A single person can make a profound difference in the world, but it is hard to transform healthcare delivery alone. A team and organizational commitment are required, but not even a team of senior leaders can mandate successful transformation—people at all levels of the organization need to be engaged. Moreover, it requires an organizational appreciation of the road ahead. The road leads to better value for patients, providers, payers, businesses, and communities

The methods and principles presented here have proven successful in navigating the changing landscape of healthcare delivery management for 20-plus years and in multiple settings. Measuring outcomes that matter to patients, implementing a systematic approach to improving those outcomes, using data responsibly, rigorously, with a fast and frugal hand, and applying leadership to govern and scale success—this is the type of healthcare system I and most of my students would design, if able to start from scratch.

CONCLUSION

What type of practice transformation will you chart? The lessons learned from decades of measuring outcomes that matter to patients provide a course for you to navigate your own course toward greater value. Change is an opportunity that does not have to be daunting. You do not have to rebuild your organization from the ground up. Everything you need is at hand, so get started now. Create an environment where you measure and act outcomes that matter to patients, and where you learn from your patients and one another as you go. The value that results will quickly become apparent to everyone who touches or is touched by your organization, inside and out. And that is how you know you are getting there.

AFTERWORD

ACKNOWLEDGEMENTS AND THANKS

I enjoy reading acknowledgments and have often noted how a book is the product of many people and a loving family that tolerated the effort. In writing this book, I learned the true depth of the words authors choose to give thanks to the people who may not have written but have endured the writer.

And I now know that merely reading the words in an acknowledgment section is like hearing parenting advice before your first child. "Your child is going to change your life," they say. You hear it and you believe it, but you do not know the sagacity of those words until you have spent time struggling to raise a child. Similarly, you only learn the true measure of the grateful words written for mentors, colleagues, and family in a book after you have spent time struggling to deliver the book.

Many mentors, colleagues, and students have shaped my career in healthcare and my thoughts on navigating towards value. I would have never started this journey without Jim Maroney's guidance and counsel. Robin McKenzie unwittingly introduced me to the use of patient reported outcomes at the point of care. James Weinstein inspired my academic efforts. Paul Batalden believed in me when I needed it most. Ano Lobb and Paul Barr brought an enviable creativity to many discussions and challenged my thinking.

John Wood, Tim Link, Craig Westling, Jeff Alderman, and Matt Grimes each read early drafts of this manuscript when it was, at best, painful to do so. They offered critical insights, constructive criticism, and continual encouragement. Chris Trimble encouraged me to go beyond sharing my research and to also tell my story. Lee Reeder provided helpful advice regarding the overall structure and flow of the manuscript. Craig Wiberg, Keith Olexa, and Peter Wacks from MGMA also provided good insight and clarifying edits.

Writing has been something I do when my daily work is done. It helps me to organize my thoughts and improves my ability to teach, but doing it means I have spent time writing when someone else might have chosen to spend time with his family. Ada and Amy, you have tolerated my choices and you each possess a work ethic that continues to inspire me. Makeda and Ethan, I know you like to profess some pride in my efforts while somewhere deep inside you still cannot believe I have gotten this far. Gannon, GMan, I have loved you from the very moment we met.

BIBLIOGRAPHY:
REFERENCES &
SUGGESTED FURTHER
READINGS

Barr, P.J., Thompson, R., Walsh, T., Grande, S.W., Ozanne, E., & Elwyn, G. (2014 Jan 3) The Psychometric Properties of CollaboRATE. A Fast and Frugal Patient Reported Measure of Shared Decision-Making Process. *Journal of Medical Internet Research*. Vol 16, No. 1

Batalden, P. *Leading the improvement of healthcare*. Retrieved March 14 2017 http://www.sheffieldmca.org.uk/UserFiles/File/Batalden_1_page_book_1.pdf

Beckhard, R., Harris R.T. (1987) *Organizational Transitions (2nd Ed)*. Reading, MA: Addison-Wesley Publishing

Berwick, W., R. Matthews, & Scanlon, C. (2010). *Achieving clinical and operational excellence: how to establish healthcare service line costs*. Redwood Shores, CA: Oracle Corp

Black, N. (2013). Patient reported outcome measures could help transform healthcare. *British Medical Journal*. 346:f167

Bohmer, R.M.J. (2010). Fixing health care on the front lines. *Harvard Business Review*. 88, 4, 62-69

Bradley, E.H., & Taylor L.A., (2013). *The American health care paradox: Why spending more is getting us less*. New York, NY: PublicAffairs

Brownlee, S. (2007). *Overtreated: Why too much medicine is making us sicker and poorer*. New York, NY: Bloomsbury USA

Brownlee, S., Colucci, J., & Walsh, T. (2012 Dec) What "health care costs" really means. *The Atlantic Magazine*. Retrieved March 14 2017 http://www.theatlantic.com/health/archive/2012/12/what-health-care-costs-really-means/266522/

Camden Coalition of Healthcare Providers (2013) *Building a hotspotting analytic toolkit*. Retrieved March 14 2017 http://www.camdenhealth.org/building-a-hotspotting-toolkit/

Butler, A.C., Chapman J.E., Forman E.M., & Beck A.T. (2006). The empirical status of cognitive-behavioral therapy: A review of meta-analyses. *Clinical Psychology Review*. 23(1), 17-31

Cady, S.H., Jacobs, J., Koller, R., & Spalding, J. (2014). The Change Formula. *OD Practitioner*. 46(3), 32-39

Carey, R. (2003) *Improving healthcare with control charts: basic and advanced SPC methods and case studies*. Milwaukee: ASQ Quality Press

Carey, R.G., & Lloyd, R.C. (2001) *Measuring Quality Improvement in Healthcare – A guide to statistical process control applications*. Milwaukee, WI: Quality Press

Collins, C., Hewson D.L., Munger, R., & Wade, T. (2010). *Evolving models of behavioral health integration in primary care*. New York, NY: The Milbank Memorial Fund

Cosgrove, D., et.al. (2012). *A CEO checklist for high value health care*. Washington, DC: Institute of Medicine

Dannemiller, K.D., & Jacobs, R.W. (1992) Changing the way organizations change. *The Journal of Applied Behavioral Science*, 28(4), 480-498

Drain, M., & Kaldenberg, D.O. (1999). Building patient loyalty and trust: The role of patient satisfaction. *Group Practice Journal*. 48(9), 32-35

Driessen, E., & Hollon, S.D. (2010). *Cognitive behavioral therapy for mood disorders: Efficacy, moderators and mediators*. The Psychiatric Clinics of North America, 33(3), 537–555. doi:10.1016/j.psc.2010.04.005

Durand, M.A., Walsh, T., Barr, P.J., Elwyn, G. (2014) Incentiving shared decision making in the USA – Where are we now?" Healthcare. Available online November 21, 2014. doi:10.1016/j.hjdsi.2014.10.008

Edwards, A. & Elwyn G. *Shared decision making in health care. Achieving evidence based patient choice*. Oxford, U.K., Oxford University Press

Elwyn, G., Barr, P.J., Grande, S.W., Walsh, T., Thompson, R., & Ozanne, E. (2013) Developing CollaboRATE. A fast and frugal measure of shared decision making in clinical encounters. *Patient Education and Counseling*. 93(1), 102-7

Elwyn, G., Lloyd, A., May, C., van der Weijden, T., Stiggelbout, A., Edwards, A., Frosch, D.L., Rapley, T., Barr, P.J., Walsh, T., Grande, S.W., Montori, V., & Epstein, R. (2014). Collaborative deliberation: A model for patient care. *Patient Education and Counseling*. 97(2), 158-164

Elwyn, G., Thompson, R., John, R., & Grande, S. (2015 March) Developing IntegRATE: a fast and frugal patient-reported measure of integration in healthcare delivery. *International Journal of Integrated Care*. 15.

Finkler, S., Ward, D., & Baker, J. (2007), *Essentials of Cost Accounting for Healthcare Organizations, 3rd ed.* Sudbury, Massachusetts: Jones and Bartlett

Frakt, A. (2014) The end of hospital cost shifting and the quest for hospital productivity. *Health Services Research*. 49(1), 1-10

Frosch, D.L., May, S.G., & Rendle, K.A.S. (May 2012). Authoritarian physicians and patients fear of being labeled 'difficult' among key obstacles to shared decision making. *Health Affairs*. 31, 51030-1038

Fussell, C.L., Hough, T. & Pedersen, M.D. (2009) *What Makes Fusion Cells Effective?* Monterey, CA: Naval Postgraduate School

Gapenski, L., (2011) *Healthcare Finance: An introduction to accounting and financial management. 4th ed.*, Chicago, IL: Health Administration Press

Gervais, M., Levant, Y. & Ducrocq, C. (2010). Time-Driven Activity-Based Costing: an initial appraisal through a longitudinal case study. *Journal of Applied Management Accounting Research*. 8(2), 1-20

Gittell, J.H., Fairfield K.M., Bierbaum, B., Head, W., Jackson, R., Kelly, M., Laskin, R., Lipson, S., Siliski J., Thornhill, T., & Zuckerman, J. (2000). Impact of Relational Coordination on Quality of Care, Postoperative Pain and Functioning and Length of Stay: A Nine-Hospital Study of Surgical Patients. *Medical Care.* 38(8), 807-819

Glover, J.A. (2008). The incidence of tonsillectomy in school children. Proceedings of the Royal Society of Medicine, 1938.31, 1219-36. *Reprinted International Journal of Epidemiology*, 37, 9-19

Goldsmith J., Burns, L.R., Sen, A., & Goldsmith, T. (2015) *Integrated delivery networks: In search of benefits and market effects.* Washington, DC: The National Academy of Social Insurance

Government Accountability Office. (2013 April). *State and local governments' fiscal outlook: April 2013 update.* Retrieved March 14 2017 http://www.gao.gov/special.pubs/longterm/state/index.html

Gravel, K., Legare, F., & Graham, I.D. (August 2006) Barriers and facilitators to implementing shared decision making clinical practice: a systematic review of health professionals' perceptions. *Implementation Science.* doi:10.1 186/1748-5908-1-16

Green,S.M., Reid, R.J., & Larson, E.B. Implementing the learning health system: From concept to action. *Annals of Internal Medicine*, 157, 207-210

Ham, C. (2010). The ten characteristics of the high-performing chronic care system. *Health Economics, Policy and Law.* 2010. 5(1), 71–9

Hawker, G.A., Wright, J.G., Coyte, P.C., Williams, J.I., Harvey, B., Glazier, R., Wilkins, A., & Badley, E.M. (2001). 'Determining the need for hip and knee arthroplasty: the role of clinical severity and patients' preferences'. *Medical Care*, 39(3), 206–16

Higgins, A., et al. (2011). Early lessons from Accountable Care Models in the private sector: Partnerships between health plans and providers. *Health Affairs, 2011.* 30(9), 1718-1727

Holdren, J.P. & Lander, E.S. (Co-Chairs). (May 2014) Better health care and lower costs: Accelerating improvement through systems engineering. *President's Council of Advisors on Science and Technology*

The Robert Wood Johnson Foundation. *How "Hot Spotting" Cut Health Care Costs*. Retrieved March 14 2017 http://www.rwjf.org/en/about-rwjf/newsroom/features-and-articles/Brenner11.html

Institute for Healthcare Improvement. *Run Chart Tool*. Retrieved March 14 2017 http://www.ihi.org/knowledge/Pages/Tools/RunChart.aspx

James, B.C., Savitz, L.A. (2011). How Intermountain trimmed health care costs through robust quality improvement efforts. *Health Affairs*, 30(6), 1185-1191

Robert Wood Johnson Foundation. *Jeff Brenner's Approach to Improving Health Care Delivery*. Retrieved March 14 2017 https://www.youtube.com/watch?v=id06Y-P58UE

Jha, A.K., & Epstein, A.M. (2009). Hospital governance and the quality of care. *Health Affairs*. doi: 10.1377/hlthaff.2009.0297

Joosten, E.A.G., DeFuentes-Merillas, L., de Weert, G.H., Sensky, T., van der Staak, C.P.F., & de Jong C.A.J. (2008). Systematic review of the effects of shared decision making on patient satisfaction, treatment adherence, and health status. *Psychotherapy and Psychosomatics*. Karger Publishers. 77, 219-226

Kaplan, G., G. Bo-Linn, P. Carayon, P. Pronovost, W. Rouse, P. Reid, &. Saunders, R. (2013). Bringing a systems approach to health. Discussion Paper, *Institute of Medicine and National Academy of Engineering, Washington, DC*. Retrieved March 14 2017 http://www.iom.edu/systemsapproaches

Kaplan, R. & Porter, M. (2011 September) How to solve the cost crisis in health care. *Harvard Business Review*

Kaplan, R.S. (May 2014). *Introduction to Time-Driven Activity-Based Costing in Healthcare.* Presented in Dublin, Ireland. Retrieved March 14 2017 http://hse.ie/eng/services/news/newsfeatures/masterclass/programme/CostMeasurement.pdf

Kotter, J. P. (2007). Leading change: Why transformation efforts fail. *Harvard Business Review*, 92, 107

Laderman, M., & Mate, K. (2014) Integrating behavioral health into Primary Care. *Healthcare Executive.* 29(2), 74-77.

Lee, C.N., Dominik R., Levin, C.A., Barry, M.J., Cosenza, C., O'Connor, A.M., Mulley, A.G. Jr., & Sepucha, K.R. (2010). Development of instruments to measure the quality of breast cancer treatment decisions. *Health Expectations*, 13(3), 258–72. doi:10.1111/j.1369-7625.2010.00600.x

Lee, C.N., Dominik, R., Levin, C.A., Barry, M.J., Cosenza, C., O'Connor, A.M., Mulley, A.G. Jr, & Sepucha, K.R. (2010). Development of instruments to measure the quality of breast cancer treatment decisions. *Health Expectations.* 13(3), 258–72. doi:10.1111/j.1369-7625.2010.00600.x

Lee, T.H. (2010). Putting the value framework to work. *New England Journal of Medicine.* 363, 2481-3

McEvoy, P., Escott, D., & Bee, P (2011). Case Management for high-intensity service users: toward a relational approach to care coordination. *Health and Social Care in the Community.* 19(1) 60 – 69

Nelson, E.C., Batalden, P., Godfrey, M.M., & Lazar, J.S. (2011). *Value by Design.* San Francisco, CA: Jossey-Bass

Nelson, E.C., Batalden, P.B., & Godfrey, M.M. (2007). *Quality by Design.* San Francisco, CA: Jossey-Bass

Nelson, L., (2012). *Lessons from Medicare's Demonstration Projects on Disease Management, Care Coordination, and Value-Based Payment.* Washington, DC: Congressional Budget Office

Nelson, W.A., Taylor, E., & Walsh, T. (2014) Leadership and transition: Building an ethical organizational culture. *The Health Care Manager.* 33, 3

Newhouse, J., & Graber, A. (Eds). (2013) *Variation in healthcare spending: Target decision making, not geography.* Washington, DC: Institute of Medicine. National Acadamies Press

Porter M.E. & Teisberg E.O. (2006). *Redefining health care: creating value-based competition on results.* Boston: Harvard Business Review Press.

Porter M.E. (2010). What is value in health care? *New England Journal of Medicine* 363, 2477-81.

Quinn, J.B. (1992) *Intelligent Enterprise.* New York, NY: Free Press

Ravallion, M. (2001). The mystery of the vanishing benefits: An introduction to impact evaluation. *The World Bank Economic Review 2001.* 15(1),115-140

Reinhardt, U. (2012 January) Divid et impera: Protecting the growth of health care incomes (costs). *Health Economics.* 21, 41-54

Rubin, H.R., et al. (1993) Patients' ratings of outpatient visits in different practice settings: Results from the Medical Outcomes Study." *Journal of the American Medical Association.* 270(7), 835-840.)

Singer, S.J., Burgers, J., Friedberg, M, Rosenthal, M.B., Leape, L., & Schneider, E. (2011) Defining and measuring integrated patient care: promoting the next frontier in health care delivery. *Medical Care Research and Review.* 68(1):112–27

Smith, M., Saunders, R., Stuckhardt., L., McGinnis, J.M. (2012). *Best care at lower cost: the path to continuously learning health care in America.* Committee on the Learning Health Care System in America. Washington DC: Institute of Medicine

Stensland, J., Gaumer Z.R., & Miller M.E. (2010) Private-payer profits can induce negative Medicare margins. *Health Affairs 2010*. 29(5),1045-1051.

Stewart, A.L., & Ware, J.E. (Eds). (1992) *Measuring functioning and well-being: The Medical Outcomes Study Approach*. Durham, NC: Duke University Press.

The Center for Medicare & Medicaid Innovation. *Priority measures for monitoring and evaluation*. Retrieved March 14 2017 http://innovation. cms.gov/Files/x/PriorityMsrMontEval.pdf

The Massachusetts Heath Policy Commission. (2013). *2013 Cost trend report*. Retrieved March 14 2017 http://www.mass.gov/anf/docs/ hpc/2013-cost-trends-report-final.pdf

Thor, J., Lundberg, J., Ask, J., Olsson J,. Carli, C., Harenstam, K.P., & Brommels, M. Application of statistical process control in healthcare: A systematic review. *Quality and Safety in Health Care*.16, 387-399

Uijen, A.A., Heinst, C.W., Schellevis, F.G., van den Bosch, W.J.H.M., van de Laar, F.A., Terwee, C.B., et al. (2012). Measurement properties of questionnaires measuring continuity of care: a systematic review. *PLoS One*. 7(7), e42256

Uijen, A.A., Schers, H.J., van Weel, C. (2013) Continuity of care preferably measured from the patients' perspective. *Journal of Clinical Epidemiology*. 63(9), 998–9.

Useem, M. (2001) *Leading Up*. New York, NY: Three Rivers Press.

Vest, J.R., & Gamm, L.D. (2009). A critical review of the research literature on six sigma, lean, and Studer Group's hardwiring excellence in the United States: The need to demonstrate and communicate the effectiveness of transformation strategies in healthcare. *Implementation Science*. 4, 35.

Walsh T., Hanscom B., Lurie J.D., & Weinstein J.N. (2003). Is a condition-specific instrument for patients with low back pain/leg symptoms really necessary? The responsiveness of the Oswestry Disability Index, MODEMS, and the SF-36. *The Spine Journal.* 15(28m), 6, 607-615.

Walsh, T., Hanscom, B., Homa, K., & Abdu, W.A. (2005) The rate and variation of referrals to behavioral medicine services for patients reporting poor mental health in the National Spine Network. *The Spine Journal.* 30(6), E154-E160.

Walsh, T., Homa, K., Lurie, J., et al. (2006). Detecting depression in patients with chronic spinal pain using the SF-36 health survey. *The Spine Journal.* (6), 16-320.

Walsh. T. & Nelson, W.A. (2014) Ensuring patient-centered care. *The Healthcare Executive.* 29, 4.

Ware, J.E., & Sherbourne, C.D. (1992). The MOS 36-item short-form health survey (SF-36): I. Conceptual framework and item selection. *Medical Care*, 30, 473-483.

Weinstein, J.N., Brown, P.W., Hanscom, B., Walsh ,T., & Nelson, E. (2000). Designing an ambulatory clinical practice for outcomes improvement: From vision to reality, The Spine Center at Dartmouth-Hitchcock, year one. *Quality Management Health Care.* 8(2), 1-20.

Welch, H.G., Schwartz, L.M., & Woloshin, S. (2011) *Overdiagnosed: Making people sick in pursuit of health.* Boston, MA: Beacon Press.

Wennberg, J.E. (2010). *Tracking Medicine: A researcher's quest to understand healthcare.* Oxford, U.K.: Oxford University Press.

White, H. (2006). *Impact Evaluation. The experience of the independent evaluation group of the World Bank.* Washington, DC: World Bank.

ABOUT THE AUTHOR;

THOM WALSH, PHD

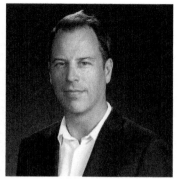

Thom is a co-founder of Cardinal Point Healthcare. Known as an excellent teacher and mentor, he draws on extensive clinical, research, and consulting experience to help people and organizations create greater value in healthcare.

His clinical career as an Orthopedic Physical Therapist spanned private practice and academic settings, including the development and launch of a multidisciplinary spine center at Dartmouth-Hitchcock Medical Center. He earned a Ph.D in Health Policy from The Dartmouth Institute for Health Policy and Clinical Practice, where he continues to teach.

His writing on ethical leadership, patient-reported outcome measures, healthcare costs and utilization, and shared decision making has appeared in numerous publications, including the BMJ, JAMA, Spine, The Journal of Healthcare Management, Forbes, The New America Foundation, and The Atlantic. Thom also enjoys ultramarathon trail races and volunteers with a search and rescue unit in the Los Angeles County Sheriff's department.

MGMA Publishing; Related Titles

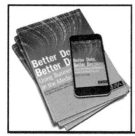

Better Data, Better Decisions: *Using Business Intelligence in the Medical Practice* demonstrates creative uses of data and reveals inexpensive data extrapolation tools, more efficient uses of data and inexpensive tools that will reduce operating costs.

mgma.com/bdbd

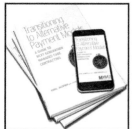

Transitioning to Alternative Payment Models helps modern practices develop a clear understanding of value based reimbursement models and how they integrate within a practice's ecosystem to increase profitability.

mgma.com/tapm

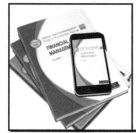

The Body of Knowledge Review Series, 3rd Edition is the seminal body of work which helps practice management professionals design and maintain efficient and effective operations that support the delivery of patient-centered care.

mgma.com/bokrs

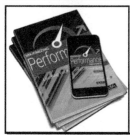

Maximizing Performance Management teaches techniques to enchance team member performance, setting expectations, planning and delegating work, rating employee performance, developing the capacity to improve employee performance and rewarding the great performances of hard-working employees.

mgma.com/mpm

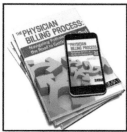

The Physician Billing Process is business critical whether you're new to medical revenue cycle management or a seasoned medical billing professional. As the medical reimbursement landscape changes, let industry experts Deborah Walker Keegan and Elizabeth Woodcock be your guides as you navigate the complex revenue cycle management journey of your medical practice.

mgma.com/pbp

CPSIA information can be obtained
at www.ICGtesting.com
Printed in the USA
LVOW05s0705220417
531742LV00008B/32/P